Hippocrasy

RACHELLE BUCHBINDER is a physician specialising in rheumatology, Director of the Monash-Cabrini Department of Musculoskeletal Health and Clinical Epidemiology at Cabrini Hospital and a Professor of Clinical Epidemiology at Monash University. She is known internationally as a vocal proponent of evidencebased medicine and for her landmark studies, particularly those examining treatments accepted into practice before proper evaluation. She has published more than 600 scientific papers and is in the top 0.1 per cent of the world's most cited scientists. She was appointed an Officer of the Order of Australia (AO) for services to epidemiology and rheumatology in 2020, and admitted as a fellow to the Australian Academy of Health and Medical Sciences in 2015.

IAN HARRIS is an orthopaedic surgeon at Liverpool, St George and Sutherland hospitals, Professor of Orthopaedic Surgery at UNSW Sydney and an Honorary Professor at the University of Sydney. Known internationally for his research and his support of evidence based practice, he has led many surgical trials and published approximately 300 scientific papers. His work has highlighted the lack of evidence for many of the treatments used in medicine, and surgery in particular, including his previous book, *Surgery, The Ultimate Placebo*, published in 2016. He was appointed a Member of the Order of Australia (AM) for services to orthopaedic surgery in 2015, and admitted as a fellow to the Australian Academy of Health and Medical Sciences in 2016.

One of the hardest things for a doctor to do ... is nothing. This superb book explains how in medicine and surgery less is often not just more, it's closer to the oath we're all supposed to practise by.

Norman Swan, award-winning producer and broadcaster of the Health Report *and* Coronacast

This eye-opening and enthralling book on the medical and moral hazards which beset the health profession is a must-read for patients and practitioners alike. From 'tooth-fairy science' to medical disasters to the inflated business world of medicine, *Hippocrasy* is a profoundly thought-provoking and compelling work that challenges our perception of the practice of modern medicine.

Kate McClymont AM, award-winning investigative journalist for the Sydney Morning Herald/The Age

Doctors are educated to do good. Yet, as the commercial imperatives of the medical industrial complex tighten their grip, doctors are becoming more and more worried that they are inflicting harm rather than creating benefit. This book is for them and, perhaps even more importantly, for their patients. The road to hell is paved with good intentions: read *Hippocrasy* and turn back.

Iona Heath CBE, former President, The Royal College of General Practitioners

This brilliant book offers clear and compelling evidence that we're all at risk from too much medicine. Using the best of science, these two respected doctors blow the whistle on harmful healthcare. Buchbinder and Harris reveal how overdiagnosis, overtreatment and the medicalisation of normal life are major threats to human health. But this brilliant book also brings hope that we can wind back the harm and waste of unnecessary tests and treatments, and focus more on the great benefits medicine has to offer.

Ray Moynihan, author of Too Much Medicine? *and* Selling Sickness, *Assistant Professor, Bond University*

About half of us in advantaged countries are now patients or 'providers', or both, and a third of clinical interventions are futile at best. Seeking health is daunting and we could benefit from a guide. Rachelle Buchbinder and Ian Harris have provided such with this volume.

Nortin M Hadler, author of The Last Well Person, The Citizen Patient *and* Worried Sick, *Emeritus Professor of Medicine and Microbiology/Immunology, University of North Carolina*

Throughout medical history, doctors have routinely ignored the fundamental Hippocratic injunction: 'First, do no harm'. Most of their treatments produced lots of harms, with little or no benefit. This wonderful book punctures the hyped claims of modern medicine, showing that it is not nearly as scientific, safe, effective, and honest as it should be. Reading *Hippocrasy* is essential for doctors (to help make them become more cautious); but even more essential for patients (to help them become more self-protective).

Allen Frances, author of Saving Normal, *Professor and Chairman Emeritus of the Department of Psychiatry and Behavioral Sciences, Duke University School of Medicine*

A timely book from two leading doctors. They present evidence that despite medicine's lip-service to evidence-based medicine, many unnecessary, wasteful and harmful investigations and treatments abound. Increasingly, the healthy are re-defined as having 'pre-disease' and drawn into questionable investigations and monitoring programmes. The book's core message is that medicine's hubris and a creeping scientism has come to overshadow the doctor's commitment to care for and comfort their patients and, above all, do no harm. It is time to step back from the brink and revisit the founding principles and core values of our profession.

Trish Greenhalgh OBE, Professor of Primary Care Research, University of Oxford

This book is dedicated to our parents,
without whom we would not have had the
opportunity, motivation or ability to write this book,
as well as to those who search for knowledge,
rather than assume it.

Hippocrasy

How doctors are betraying their oath

**Rachelle Buchbinder
and Ian Harris**

NEWSOUTH

A NewSouth book

Published by
NewSouth Publishing
University of New South Wales Press Ltd
University of New South Wales
Sydney NSW 2052
AUSTRALIA
newsouthpublishing.com

A catalogue record for this book is available from the National Library of Australia

ISBN   9781742237350 (paperback)
         9781742238265 (ebook)
         9781742239156 (ePDF)

Internal design Josephine Pajor-Markus
Cover design Peter Long
Cover image Shutterstock
Printer Griffin Press, part of Ovato

Contents

The Hippocratic Oath

Modern version by Louis Lasagna, 1964

I swear to fulfil, to the best of my ability and judgment, this covenant:

- I will respect the hard-won scientific gains of those physicians in whose steps I walk, and gladly share such knowledge as is mine with those who are to follow.
- I will apply, for the benefit of the sick, all measures which are required, avoiding those twin traps of overtreatment and therapeutic nihilism.
- I will remember that there is art to medicine as well as science, and that warmth, sympathy, and understanding may outweigh the surgeon's knife or the chemist's drug.
- I will not be ashamed to say 'I know not', nor will I fail to call in my colleagues when the skills of another are needed for a patient's recovery.
- I will respect the privacy of my patients, for their problems are not disclosed to me that the world may know. Most especially must I tread with care in matters of life and death. If it is given me to save a life, all thanks. But it may also be within my power to take a life; this awesome responsibility must be faced with great humbleness and awareness of my own frailty. Above all, I must not play at God.
- I will remember that I do not treat a fever chart, a cancerous growth, but a sick human being, whose illness may affect

the person's family and economic stability. My responsibility includes these related problems, if I am to care adequately for the sick.

- I will prevent disease whenever I can, for prevention is preferable to cure.
- I will remember that I remain a member of society, with special obligations to all my fellow human beings, those sound of mind and body as well as the infirm.
- If I do not violate this oath, may I enjoy life and art, respected while I live and remembered with affection thereafter. May I always act so as to preserve the finest traditions of my calling and may I long experience the joy of healing those who seek my help.

Introduction

While many medical students take the Hippocratic Oath or a similar pledge before graduating (reciting lines like first, do no harm) we've ended up with a healthcare system that's one of the greatest threats to human health. Our own experience as doctors and researchers has shown that much of medicine doesn't do what it's supposed to do: improve health. Modern medical care is designed to maximise the number of encounters with the system, constantly prescribing, operating, testing and scanning, and prioritising business over science. It's a system rife with perverse incentives and unintended consequences, producing health care without necessarily improving the health of the recipients of that care. The problem threatens the delivery of efficient and effective health care, wastes money and causes harm.

We're both doctors in the field of musculoskeletal medicine. Ian is an orthopaedic surgeon and Rachelle is a rheumatologist. We're also internationally acclaimed academics in science-based medicine. In our research, our aim is to determine the true value of specific medical practices, which is often very different from their *perceived* value. We're both highly published professors: between us we've published about a thousand scientific and lay articles. Ian has also written a popular book, *Surgery, The Ultimate Placebo*, which exposed the lack of effectiveness of many surgical procedures. *Hippocrasy* goes further by looking at medicine as a whole, from birth to death. It's informed as much by our clinical work caring for individual patients as by our academic work.

The more we see of medicine and the way it's practised, and the more we learn from our research and the research of others, the more we're convinced that doctors are getting it wrong. Doctors commonly overtreat, the harms of treatment go under-reported or under-recognised, and they often ignore or misunderstand the science, or don't know it in the first place. And these problems are driven by the personal biases of the doctors themselves.

We trained under a system of apprenticeship, learning from the examples of others, assuming it was the right thing to do. It was only later, after we learned the skills of critical thinking and science, that we realised much of what we were doing was useless, harmful or both. We realised that doctors should look at medicine as any good scientist would look at a subject, by recognising and putting aside personal biases and questioning the current thinking using unbiased (scientific) methods.

Our training and working careers never overlapped but took very similar trajectories. After completing training in our specialist fields, we began to question the standard practices advised by our teachers. We both undertook Masters degrees in evidence-based medicine (clinical epidemiology) and later doctoral degrees in the same field. This further training reinforced our scepticism of modern medicine and provided us with the scientific tools to answer many of the questions we were asking. We began studying the effectiveness of common treatments and speaking out against what we saw as the harmful and wasteful use of ineffective treatments. Inevitably this led to us crossing paths, initially briefly when attending the same conferences, but most notably at the second international Preventing Overdiagnosis Conference in Oxford in 2014, where our alliance was forged. Since then, we have worked closely together on academic pursuits, including many successful grants, trials, guidelines and other projects.

We're not alone in experiencing such an epiphany – many people have written about the harms and overtreatment rife in modern medicine. Leading medical journals and global movements have taken on the challenge of overtreatment, medical harm, overdiagnosis and the medicalisation of 'normal'. For example, the *British Medical Journal* (with 'Too Much Medicine') and the *Journal of the American Medical Association* ('Less Is More') have regular sections devoted to tackling the problem. Choosing Wisely, a clinician-led initiative that identifies the top five tests, treatments or procedures doctors and patients should question within each field of medicine, now has national branches in many countries. International meetings such as the annual Preventing Overdiagnosis Conference, and networks of like-minded doctors and other healthcare professionals, academics and consumers, such as the Australian Wiser Healthcare collaboration, specifically address the issues raised in this book. Unfortunately, these concepts haven't broken through to become common knowledge or accepted by everyone – doctors and general public alike.

We're not suggesting for a minute that doctors are malicious or deliberately advising ineffective or harmful treatments. Many doctors remain unaware of the criticisms and continue to act *in good faith* while contributing to the problem. We're suggesting that doctors who base their practices on what's commonly accepted, or on what they perceive to be effective, are often, unknowingly, wrong. And that's bad for everyone.

Most people cling to the tradition that if a doctor recommends something then it must be good and we should act on their advice. How is it, then, that doctors differ so widely in their opinions? Why are they so likely to recommend treatments provided by their own specialty, yet talk down the treatments provided by others? Why is medical care, in itself, often listed as a leading cause of death? And if much of modern medicine is ineffective and harmful, why are doctors still providing it?

In *Hippocrasy*, we will use the Hippocratic Oath (see pages ix–x) – the series of pledges commonly considered to be the ethical basis and guiding framework for the practice of medicine – to answer these questions and more. We will show you how the medical community is betraying the ideal that the Oath represents.

Medicine's betrayal of the ideals of the Hippocratic Oath is expressed in many ways: in unnecessary health care, in our overdependence on medicine in our daily life, and in the direct and indirect personal harms suffered by those who place their trust in medicine. Furthermore, this betrayal has come at great cost: the focus on unnecessary, expensive and ineffective tests and treatments has diverted our efforts and resources away from providing effective care to those who truly need it.

Doctors are rarely blamed for the problems with medicine, despite being in charge of much of it and being in a position to change things for the better. While unnecessary treatment is a big issue, many are reluctant to blame those performing the needless operations, writing the unnecessary prescriptions, and taking the incentives – the doctors themselves. Instead, 'the system' is blamed.

Medicine versus public health measures

Doctors (and modern medicine) are generally held in high regard, yet you might be surprised to learn that much of the success of modern medicine is more apparent than real. Most of the major advances in health and life expectancy over the past couple of hundred years weren't due to modern medicine, but to public health, political and industrial achievements, such as clean water supply, sewerage separation, having enough food and avoiding war. Despite the enormous benefits that public health measures have brought, societies spend most of their resources on individualised health care – care that emphasises technological advances and expensive treatments rather than focusing on public health programs and other preventive strategies that are likely to have far greater positive impacts on health. Obesity, for example, is seen as a major contributor to poor health and high health costs due to its association with type 2 diabetes, heart disease, cancer and arthritis, to name a few. Yet rather than treating it as a public health problem, by modifying food legislation and incentives, educating the public and changing the 'obesogenic' culture to *prevent* it, the public, the doctors and other healthcare providers are focused on high-risk, high-cost medical treatments – such as gastric surgery, which provides inconsistent results.

Medical care has not universally or consistently improved health or quality of life. There are, of course, highly successful medical therapies, such as chemotherapy for childhood leukaemias, which have saved lives; and hip replacement and cataract surgery, which have improved quality of life for millions. But many other medical interventions, despite having proven ineffective and even harmful, remain in common use. Astoundingly, it has been estimated that *about one-third of medical care is of no value, while another 10 per cent is actually harmful.*

Yet despite widespread evidence of this, much of which is discussed in this book, many doctors continue to perform procedures and prescribe treatments known to be ineffective. Even when unhelpful or harmful practices have declined, it has usually taken many years, often decades. For example, arthroscopy to treat painful knees due to wear and tear was first found to be ineffective almost 20 years ago, but its use only started waning about a decade ago, and in some places hasn't declined at all.

Many factors contribute to the failure to abandon ineffective medical practices, from ingrained and difficult-to-shift beliefs about their perceived effectiveness, to the conviction that doing something is better than doing nothing. While most people would agree that we should be cautious about introducing new medical advances into routine medical practice before they have been properly evaluated, we repeatedly fail to do so. Although driven by the well-intentioned desire to pass on the presumed benefits to society that new advances in treatment promise, their rapid introduction into routine care often backfires. Not only may the benefits be overestimated, but the harms may only become evident once those treatments have been introduced.

Since we started writing this book, the world has experienced the COVID-19 pandemic. In the early days, doctors and others were touting the benefits of the so-called miracle drug hydroxychloroquine, an effective antimalarial medication also commonly used to treat autoimmune diseases such as rheumatoid arthritis and systemic lupus erythematosus (better known as lupus). It began being prescribed in large numbers to people with the virus. Australian doctors also started prescribing the drug for themselves and their family members as a 'preventive' measure. Despite the hype associated with the very early preliminary studies, however, it was subsequently found to be ineffective against COVID, with a risk of significant life-threatening side effects.

While many worthy efforts were directed towards finding effective and safe vaccines and identifying and evaluating promising life-saving treatments, the pandemic has highlighted many of the issues we describe in this book. Of all the widespread touting of drugs to both prevent and treat COVID-19, very few have so far been shown to be of any benefit. It has been public health measures that have been largely responsible for reducing infection rates. Countries that adopted public health measures such as working from home, social distancing, mask wearing and contact tracing have minimised the impact of the virus and, in many cases, eradicated community transmission almost completely.

Misplaced faith in premature results can also lead to other harms: in the case of hydroxychloroquine, the hype led to widespread shortages of the drug for patients, including our own, who were taking the medication for sometimes life-threatening diseases such as lupus. In Australia, the mining magnate and former politician Clive Palmer was given permission by Australia's drug regulators to import millions of doses of the drug to add to government stockpiles, adding to the worldwide shortage. The pandemic has also offered opportunities to profit from peoples' COVID fears by marketing fake treatments. Examples include the 'BioCharger' device (from chef Pete Evans) and peptides (from 'Dr Ageless', Shane Charter).

Medical harms and waste or 'low-value' care (where treatment is provided at some cost but offers no meaningful benefits) have been well documented over many years, but this message remains largely underappreciated. The default position is to believe that all medical tests and treatments are worthwhile, and the more medical care the better. Because the problem affects everyone, and because we all should have a say in how our health and our medical concerns are addressed, every one of us needs to understand these problems.

Why we wrote this book

We were motivated to write *Hippocrasy* by the daily reminders of the harms that come from society's over-reliance on medicine; the waste from performing or prescribing unnecessary, ineffective or marginally effective tests, medicines and procedures; the problems that come from treating medicine as a business; and the misdirected incentives of a medical system that doesn't necessarily work to improve health. Attempts to improve health care are also misdirected. The current worldwide 'affordability' crisis in medicine is too focused on reducing costs through economic and production-based models of care (where more care is better but needs to be more efficient), ignoring the savings that could be achieved through reducing unnecessary, wasteful and harmful medical care.

Despite the COVID-19 pandemic, there's no doubt that the biggest global health threat of the 21st century is climate change. We've recently seen stark examples of the impact of climate change on human health. This includes the unprecedented Melbourne 'thunderstorm asthma' epidemic in 2016, which resulted in 14000 people attending hospital, a 3000 per cent increase in intensive care admissions, and ten deaths. The hundreds of bushfires that ravaged south-eastern Australia over the 2019–20 summer not only claimed lives but also caused air pollution many times above hazardous levels, with 11 million people experiencing some smoke exposure, and large numbers reporting physical and/or mental symptoms. While the long-term effects are as yet unknown, evidence from other severe bushfires indicates that this is likely to include extra premature deaths and cardiovascular and respiratory events, as well as anxiety, depression, substance abuse and post-traumatic stress disorder (PTSD).

What's much less appreciated, however, is that health care *itself* damages the environment. A 2018 study published in *Lancet Planet Health* and led by Dr Forbes McGain, an Australian anaesthetist and intensive care physician as well as one of the world's leading experts on the effects of health care on the environment, estimated that health care produces about 7 per cent of Australia's total carbon emissions. To put this into perspective, this is about half the total carbon emissions of the whole Australian construction industry, including construction of all buildings, pipelines, dams, oil rigs, roads and rail lines. Reducing unnecessary, wasteful and harmful medical care makes sense for the good of the environment and the environmental sustainability of the healthcare system, as well as our health.

What to expect from this book

Let's have a brief look at some of the major themes we will explore in *Hippocrasy*.

Medicalisation

Medicalisation is the process by which 'normal' human conditions, such as sadness and grief, slightly elevated blood pressure, shyness, menopause and ageing, come to be defined (and treated) as medical conditions. Perceived 'deviations' from normal are viewed from the perspective of a simplistic medical model called the disease–illness paradigm, which implies that every 'abnormality' has a traceable, direct physical cause. In short, any departure from normal is diagnosed as an illness, and, once diagnosed, the 'illness' is subject to medical treatment. The problem, of course, lies in who gets to decide what's abnormal, what drives them to make that call, and whether it helps the people labelled as abnormal.

Medicalisation comes from the doctors themselves and the industry that supports the practice of medicine – drug and device manufacturers, hospital owners, and so on – but we're all complicit and all too willing to believe that the process is in our best interests when the opposite is often true.

Other drivers of medicalisation include society's over-reliance on the medical system to address what are simply the benign predicaments of life rather than diseases that would benefit from medical intervention. Unpleasant sensations like an ordinary headache, mild anxiety or irregular bowel habits, which were once considered a normal part of life, have become medical conditions requiring medical treatment. This has resulted in a decline in our resilience and ability to tolerate the usual ups and downs of life that create discomfort or unease. Instead, they are outsourced to the medical community, making coping a *passive* process. Yet there's consistent evidence that coping is best performed *actively* by the person with the condition, and that our ability to cope and adapt in response to challenges is a measure of our health, and therefore not something we should delegate to others.

Despite easy access to medical information from Dr Google, doctors still hold the upper hand regarding medical knowledge. This 'knowledge asymmetry' between doctors and patients is a driver of medicalisation. It produces a moral hazard in which doctors make decisions yet the burden of risk is placed on the patient. It also allows perverse incentives to prevail, whereby doctors can easily justify treatments that will benefit them financially – for example, by recommending surgery for which they will be paid, further accentuated if they also own the hospital. This biases doctors towards intervening, and makes it easy for them to make a patient believe they need the treatment.

We cover medicalisation throughout the book, and in depth in chapter 9.

Overdiagnosis

Overdiagnosis occurs when someone is given a diagnosis that's technically correct but won't benefit them and might cause harm. It can occur when healthy people are screened for diseases such as cancer, and abnormalities are detected that would not have caused any symptoms or clinical problems in their lifetime. Not only would they never have known they had the condition, but they would have lived just as long had it not been diagnosed in the first place.

Overdiagnosis can also occur when people with minor symptoms are investigated unnecessarily. A scan might show an abnormality that could be an age-related change – it's not the cause of their problem but is falsely assumed to be. Overdiagnosis occurs, too, when disease definitions are widened, officially or unofficially, resulting in people previously considered normal or within a spectrum of normal being classified as diseased.

Examples of overdiagnosis include the lowering of the threshold for hypertension (high blood pressure), osteopaenia (thin bones) and attention deficit hyperactivity disorder (ADHD). In the case of hypertension and osteopaenia, mere risk factors for disease (high blood pressure for heart failure and strokes, and thin bones for fracture) are now labelled as diseases in their own right. Overdiagnosis can also occur with the creation of new diseases, such as sarcopenia (weak muscles) and female sexual dysfunction.

In all of these cases, the diagnoses are technically correct (i.e. they're not misdiagnoses), but detecting, labelling or redefining the problem as a disease doesn't benefit the person being diagnosed. Apart from being unnecessary to the improvement of health, overdiagnosis often leads to psychological distress from being labelled, physical harms from unnecessary treatment, and financial costs to both the individual and society.

Overdiagnosis, which occurs as a result of overtesting and leads to overtreatment, is discussed throughout the book.

Overtreatment

Like overdiagnosis, overtreatment can be defined as health care (consultations, tests, drugs, procedures, and so on) that provides no benefit to the patient. It's often driven by a distorted perception of medical care that overestimates the benefits and underestimates the harms. Other factors that contribute to overtreatment are the practice of defensive medicine due to fear of litigation, health systems that incentivise tests and/or treatments rather than health improvements, and equating a failure to treat with a failure to care.

We cover overtreatment in detail in chapter 3.

Medicine as big business

Modern medical care has been packaged into a business model for which it's unsuited. Medicine doesn't obey the laws of economics: for example, the increased supply of doctors *creates* demand. Treating health care as a commodity incentivises processes over outcomes, the complex over the simple, and treatment over prevention. Furthermore, doctors (who control the spending) don't bear the cost burden of their decisions. Most importantly, if medicine becomes big business, it must work primarily to create profit. Too often, profit is derived from delivering more health care at the highest price, regardless of effectiveness or harms. The ability of large health companies to influence our medical systems towards driving profit over health may be one of the greatest threats to health.

Many doctors and academic organisations are challenging medicine from within. This book picks up that thread, explaining what's wrong with the practice of medicine and how it can be addressed.

We discuss this issue in detail in chapter 4.

What isn't in this book

We commonly find that our views on modern medicine are shared by practitioners of alternatives to medicine, and that they use our work to support their own cause. We accept the support but need to state clearly that by being critical of medicine and demanding that it be improved, we're not implying that alternatives to medicine are superior.

We deliberately avoid commenting on the benefits and harms of practices outside the field of medicine because it's simply not our aim and including them would detract from our core message that there are problems *within* medicine. We expect those outside of medicine to adhere to the same scientific and ethical principles we demand of medicine and any other profession that deals with vulnerable individuals.

Hippocrasy discusses many treatments and tests used in medicine, but this shouldn't be taken as individual medical advice. We encourage potential patients and patients who are contemplating changes in their health care to discuss any of the points raised in this book with their doctor.

The Hippocratic Oath

We believe that all doctors should aspire to uphold the principles enshrined in the Oath. By using its pledges as a focus for each chapter, we cover all the ways doctors are harming and not helping people by betraying the Oath. We use the most widely adopted version of the Hippocratic Oath, the 1964 ('modern') version written by the academic dean of the School of Medicine at Tufts University. Hippocrates (460–370BCE) is considered the father of medicine. His original Oath is no longer used today, and doesn't entirely represent the ideals enshrined in the modern version. The original Oath mainly states that doctors should respect and financially support their teacher, maintain patient privacy, not poison their patients, treat the sick and try to avoid 'injury and wrongdoing'.

Given the intention of the original Oath to avoid 'injury and wrongdoing', we have taken the liberty of including in the book, in addition to the modern version of the Oath, the commonly associated pledge: *'Primum non nocere'* ('First, do no harm').

* * *

We hope that this book will help you see medicine as we do: as an inflated business rife with biases and perverse incentives that lead to too much medicine, delivered at great cost and causing great harm; and as a system designed to deliver health care that does so often to the detriment of health. The harmful effects on health occur both at the level of the individual patient, and, via its environmental impacts, the wider population. At the very least, we hope this book will help you become more sceptical of health care and to ask the right questions of your doctors:

- Has this treatment been *proven* to work in high-quality studies?
- What were the actual results?
- Are the benefits worth the risks?
- What alternatives are there?
- What would happen if I did nothing?

1
First, do no harm

'Whenever a doctor cannot do good,
he must be kept from doing harm'
– attributed to Hippocrates

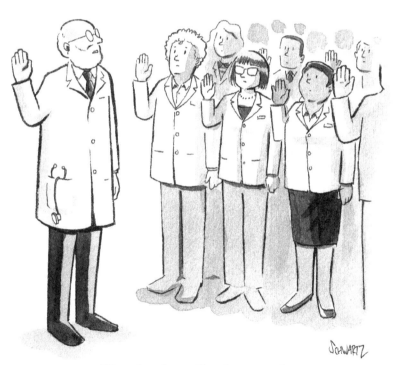

"First, do no harm. After that, go nuts."

One of Australia's worst medical scandals exemplifies the fundamental importance of the pledge 'First, do no harm'. It occurred at Chelmsford Private Hospital in a suburb of Sydney between 1963 and 1979. Over this period 'deep sleep therapy' was administered to more than a thousand people for a variety of conditions, including depression, anxiety, mania, alcoholism and heroin addiction. This occurred despite most psychiatrists having concluded that the original precursor of this treatment, pioneered in the early 20th century for 'shell shock', was both ineffective and dangerous.

At Chelmsford Hospital, patients received a cocktail of barbiturates that put them in a coma for up to two weeks, sometimes longer. They were fed through a tube into their stomach, nursed naked and unmonitored in a normal ward, and were often incontinent and constipated. They were shackled to the bed in case they woke up, and some were given electroconvulsive shock therapy without their knowledge or consent. At least 24 people died from the treatment, some within days of being admitted to the hospital, and a further 24 were alleged to have died from suicide within a year of the treatment. Hundreds of others were also harmed; they lost a considerable amount of weight, woke up confused and weak, and some developed chest and urinary infections, and blood clots.

The doctors who administered the treatment were convinced that it worked. In fact, two doctors who worked at the hospital, one of whom part-owned it, still appear to believe the treatment works. In 2020 they lost a multimillion-dollar defamation case against HarperCollins after the 2016 publication of a book called *Fair Game: The Incredible Untold Story of Scientology in Australia* by Steve Cannane. The book had referenced the doctors' role in the abuse as well as the part that Scientology had played in exposing it. The judge dismissed the case, finding that the two doctors had used the proceedings to 'rewrite history and vindicate their conduct' despite overwhelming evidence to the contrary. The damning

Chelmsford Royal Commission, which took place only after public outcry and pressure from the media, found evidence of unethical and sustained negligent medical malpractice.

This disturbing incident is emblematic of problems highlighted in this book. It's what can happen when doctors are trusted too much, by both the vulnerable patients – many of whom weren't fully informed of the treatment or the risks in this case – and the regulators. Complaints about deep sleep therapy were received over many years but weren't fully investigated. The power given to doctors in the medical system is arguably too great when episodes like this can occur without challenge, or without the challenges succeeding.

The story of deep sleep therapy also illustrates a lack of respect for science in that the treatment was introduced without any real scientific scrutiny and was then allowed to continue for more than a decade. This much more extreme form of the ineffective therapy used for shell shock was used because it *appeared* to work. There were no studies assessing whether the hypothesised benefits of an extended 'mental holiday' were real, no studies assessing its safety, and no studies comparing it to other treatments. The biased view of the observer, the doctor who invented and promoted it, Dr Harry Bailey, led to a gross overestimation of the benefits (there were none) and an underestimation of the harms (there were plenty). As the chief psychiatrist at Chelmsford at the time, Dr Bailey bore primary responsibility for the deaths. He committed suicide by taking an overdose of barbiturates while he was under investigation. Believing in the treatment to the end, he left a suicide note that stated, 'Let it be known that the Scientologists and the forces of madness have won'.

This case also illustrates how slowly practice change occurs in medicine. Even with the poor evidence available – based upon sedating soldiers with shell shock for just a few hours – most psychiatrists had already concluded that it was useless and harmful, well before the treatments were used at Chelmsford Hospital. It shows the problem with the business model of medicine and competing interests: the doctors were paid to prescribe the treatment and these treatments kept the small private hospital in business. And finally, it shows the harms that flow from medicalising conditions – such as anxiety and premenstrual stress – that may be a normal part of life.

We tend to assume that older treatments are no longer performed because they've been superseded or replaced by more effective treatments but, as in this case, treatments are often abandoned because they never worked in the first place. They were introduced based largely on the notion that they *could* work or *should* work, not that they *did* work.

The deep sleep therapy saga is also symbolic of other problems with modern medicine. Doctors, in their desire to diagnose and treat – even conditions that are better left alone – are harming people. Doctors don't *intend* to harm people: they believe that the potential benefits of their actions outweigh the potential harms. Yet they do harm people unintentionally, and in much larger numbers than you might think.

How medical care is *supposed* to work

The probabilities of benefits and harms from any particular test or treatment are calculated in studies that collectively involve many people. Usually, hundreds of people are needed to ensure these probabilities are accurate and unbiased. Smaller studies risk either finding a benefit where none exists or missing an important benefit due to chance. The larger the study, provided other potential biases have been minimised, the more faith we can have in the results. For example, thousands of patients were needed to accurately test the effectiveness of COVID vaccines – tests that were found to be accurate on wider rollout.

Doctors then use these probabilities to decide whether or not the test or treatment is suitable for an individual patient, taking into account how similar the patient is to the people in the studies. They discuss the potential benefits and harms of a proposed test or treatment with the patient, taking into consideration the patient's circumstances as well as their values and preferences. They then help the patient weigh up all this information and reach an informed decision, taking into account what's important to the patient. The treatment either pays off or it doesn't – the result is either a net benefit or a net harm. Even if it doesn't work, at least the most rational course, the one most *likely* to succeed, was taken.

How medical care *usually* works

Doctors' perceptions about the balance of benefits and risks of any type of medical intervention are often wrong. They commonly overestimate the benefits, while under-recognising and underestimating the harms. This biases the decision-making towards *more* medical care rather than *less*, resulting in excess harm and less benefit than expected. While this mightn't sound like much, this kind of bias has led to large-scale harms.

History is full of examples of treatments that were routinely used based on their perceived benefit, only to find out later that they were harming people: thalidomide to treat morning sickness in pregnant women, putting stents into blocked coronary arteries in people who have no symptoms, and arthroscopic surgery for people with knee pain.

You might think, just as past generations did, that these unfortunate errors are in the past and we've learned from them, but you'd be wrong. We continue to repeat these mistakes over and over. Many of the treatments we use today are harming patients and will be the failures the next generation identifies. What's worse, we *already know* that many of the treatments we use today provide no benefits and/or are harmful, yet we continue to use them.

As recently as 2013, researchers published a study examining more than 2000 articles on the effectiveness of medical treatments published in the leading medical journals from 2001 to 2010. Of the 363 articles testing what was considered standard practice, 40 per cent found that the standard practice did not work. All of those ineffective treatments were widely used (many still are) and all of them carry risks of harm. Examples include treating healthy postmenopausal women with hormone replacement therapy to prevent heart disease – it actually increases the risk, especially in the first year of treatment; and intensive lowering of blood sugar in people with diabetes to reduce heart attacks and strokes – intensive control has not been shown to improve mortality or cardiovascular outcomes, and at least two studies have found that it might increase the risk of dying compared with more liberal blood sugar control.

The trouble with medical harm

Despite being studied much more in recent decades, the concept of medical harm is still poorly understood by doctors, other healthcare professionals and the general public. Medical harm doesn't just refer to side effects from treatments or complications after surgery. It refers to the harms from all decisions doctors make. It can relate to diagnoses – missing a diagnosis, delaying a diagnosis or making the wrong diagnosis – and many of these issues will result in treatment errors as well, such as giving the wrong treatment (wrong medicine, wrong dose, and so on), failing to treat or giving excess treatment.

Even after the doctor has taken all known precautions, some medical harms aren't totally preventable. For example, there may be no way of predicting whether someone is going to have an allergic reaction the first time they take an antibiotic such as penicillin, and even with meticulous care, not all infections after surgery can be prevented. Preventable harms are usually only considered to be those resulting from medical errors that occur in the delivery of what's presumed to be *necessary* care – for example, giving the wrong drug or dose of drug, or accidentally operating on the wrong limb.

But this assumes that the care was justified in the first place. It's increasingly being recognised that a sizeable proportion of preventable harm is produced by *unnecessary* or *unwarranted* medical intervention – harm that could have been avoided had the test not been requested, the diagnosis never been made, or the treatment never been given in the first place.

While the medical harm that arises from mistakes in delivering care has been well studied, the medical harm from unwarranted or unnecessary care in the first place has received much less focus. Care can be considered unnecessary if the known benefits don't outweigh the known risks. It arises, for example, when a particular treatment has been proven to be no better than placebo (no treatment, but disguised so that the patient thinks they are receiving the drug or surgery) or another safer treatment, but is given anyway. An example might be developing a severe allergic reaction to an antibiotic prescribed for the common cold (for which antibiotics are neither effective nor necessary). While we're most concerned in this book about the preventable harm from unnecessary or unwarranted medical intervention, it's instructive to first explore what's known about the extent of medical harm produced by *necessary* care.

Medical errors and preventable complications

Most of the information we have on medical harm relates to medical care in hospitals. One in ten people admitted to hospital have a complication; many are preventable. A 1995 report from the US Institute of Medicine detailed the extent of medical error in

US hospitals, based on studies done in the 1980s. It concluded that between 44 000 and 98 000 people in the United States die each year as a result of medical errors occurring during hospitalisation, often in surgery, intensive care or the emergency department, or through medication errors. A later US study, using data from four studies of hospitalisations occurring from the 2000s, found the numbers were much greater. It estimated that between 210 000 and 400 000 people die each year as a result of errors during hospitalisation, while non-lethal harms (such as side effects from prescribed drugs and complications from incorrect or ineffective procedures) were estimated to be ten to 20 times more common.

Outside the United States, equivalent studies have yielded similar results. For example, the Quality in Australian Health Care Study, published in 1995, reported that 18 000 preventable deaths occur in Australia each year as a result of medical error, and more than 15 per cent of hospital admissions involve an adverse event, for example, a wound infection or blood clots after surgery. Studies from many countries put the figure for adverse events from hospital treatment at around 10 per cent. In other words, for every ten hospital admissions, we can expect one adverse event. There is, however, some variation in the proportion judged to be preventable. For example, a 2008 review of studies in the United States, Canada, the United Kingdom, Australia and New Zealand found an adverse event rate of 9.2 per cent, about half of which were preventable, while a more recent study from Ireland reported that 70 per cent of the adverse events were preventable.

The rate of harms from hospitalisation in developing countries is similar: a 2012 study of selected African and Middle Eastern nations found the rate of adverse events was 8.2 per cent, and most were considered preventable. The overall consistency of results across different studies (even considering the different methods used), makes a good argument that this isn't just a one-off finding or something only confined to one region or health system.

While the problem is large enough for one report to conclude that medical error is the third leading cause of death in the United States, this may actually be an underestimate, as medical error isn't listed as a cause of death on death certificates or in diagnostic disease listings. Another study ranked medical error at 14th in the list of conditions contributing to the global burden of disease (not just death), alongside malaria and tuberculosis. An Organisation for Economic Co-operation and Development (OECD) report involving 37 member countries highlighted the direct costs and loss of productivity resulting from these harms. A further problem is that the definition of 'preventable' is difficult – some judgment is required. For example, in sick patients, there's a risk of death regardless of what the doctors do, so determining if and how much a medical error contributed to the death can be difficult.

Although many criticisms have been levelled at studies estimating the extent of medical harm in hospitals, including their accuracy and precision, no one has denied that it's a big problem. So while we cannot say with certainty that medical error is the third (or 30th) leading cause of death, we can confidently state that it's a common cause of death and harm. On the other hand, because medical error isn't listed as a cause of death or disability in official reports, it's hard to identify and therefore hard to act on. In effect, the high rates of harm from medical error aren't being met with proportionate actions to prevent them.

Medical errors outside hospitals

Studies performed outside of hospital care also find substantial rates of medical error. For example, a population-based survey relying on the reporting of medical harm from people in the community found that more than one in five Americans have experienced a medical error in their own care, most of which occurred outside the hospital. Most commonly these were missed, incorrect or delayed diagnoses or medication errors, and most related to healthcare providers not paying attention to detail.

Medical harm from *unnecessary* care

Another reason harm from medical error doesn't attract the attention it deserves might be that it doesn't tally with our belief that doctors only do good things. It's easy (and common) to consider the harms caused by medical care as part of the price we pay to have modern medicine, and that the harms are being minimised as much as possible. Why wouldn't doctors be minimising the harms? The answer to that question is that many of them don't know the extent of the problem or don't believe it.

What if most of the harms arising from medical care are *separate* from the benefits medicine provides? What if they're not 'part of the package' or 'the price we pay' for the benefits modern medicine can undoubtedly supply? When harms such as death or life-threatening complications such as severe infection are preventable and arise from unnecessary care, this is a tragedy. It's completely avoidable and not offset by any associated benefit.

These hospital and population-based studies only examined the preventability of adverse events based on features of the care provided – were antibiotics given, was the patient checked properly for pressure areas, and so on. They didn't consider whether the care was needed in the first place. The *necessity* of treatment is rarely questioned, but both non-preventable and preventable medical errors can easily be avoided if the treatment isn't given in the first place. If there's good evidence that a treatment is no better than a placebo or sham treatment, no treatment at all or a safer treatment, then any harm resulting from that treatment can be considered avoidable. And this goes for all types of medical care or treatments, including prescription drugs, surgery, chemotherapy, radiotherapy, physical and psychological therapies, and even investigations such as blood tests and scans, or more invasive tests such as angiograms and biopsies.

The extent of unnecessary care is much higher than most people think – it isn't a small problem. The US Institute of Medicine has estimated that 30 cents of every dollar spent on health care in the United States is for unnecessary care, totalling US$750 billion annually. This is likely to be similar in Australia and many other developed countries. Given that the most common causes of in-hospital medical error are drug reactions and surgery, it's worth looking at the possible extent of overtreatment (unnecessary care) in those areas alone. This could potentially convert many of those 'non-preventable' complications into preventable ones. For example, if we could reduce or eliminate unnecessary cardiac stenting in people with heart disease, comprehensive full-body health check-ups in well people, tonsillectomies and many types of cancer screening, then this would also reduce the complications arising from them.

But wait, there's more

So far, we have considered the direct (physical) harms that can result from medical decisions. But the harm from medical decision-making extends beyond that. Medical harm also includes mental or emotional harm resulting from being treated disrespectfully, being talked down to, not having concerns taken seriously, or not being communicated with at all. These harms can result not only in dissatisfaction with care, but poorer patient health outcomes as well as a reluctance to seek medical attention in the future. There are also significant harms in labelling people with a diagnosis – converting them from a healthy person or otherwise healthy person with some complaints, to a person with a disease or disability – even if no treatment is given.

The other harm from overtreatment is the cost, particularly the opportunity costs. The time that patients, doctors and other healthcare workers devote to unnecessary care is time not spent productively. The money spent on unnecessary care is also money not spent on necessary care.

The history of medical harm

In the more than 100 years since schizophrenia has been a diagnosis, treatments have included incarceration, an array of toxic drugs such as injections of sulfur and oil, inducing fevers, praying and going to church. In 1910, Winston Churchill suggested mass sterilisation of people with severe mental illnesses such as schizophrenia.

For as long as there have been healers, there have been ineffective and harmful treatments. Sometimes the treatments were based upon mistaken beliefs about their effects and sometimes they were based on erroneous diagnoses. And, of course, there have always been charlatans. People of each era have looked back at the past and considered such treatment errors to be a product of an unenlightened time. Many have seen their own time as free from such treatment errors, but then the next age looked back on *them*. As the following examples will illustrate, however, we don't appear to have learned from our mistakes.

Bloodletting

One of the earliest and most pervasive treatments given by doctors was to bleed people. Performed in many ways, by cutting veins or using leeches (in the early 1800s, France alone was using about 60 million leeches each year for this purpose), the procedure was justified by many different theories, mainly centred on removing 'bad' things from the body. Bloodletting was used to treat a whole range of conditions, including seizures, fevers, headaches, pneumonia, haemorrhoids and even blood loss from wounds.

The harmful medical practice of removing a person's blood persisted for more than 2000 years before being seriously questioned at the beginning of the 19th century. The first clue came from observing that a decline in the practice coincided with fewer deaths from pneumonia. In 1816 a military surgeon, Alexander Lesassier Hamilton, described one of the first 'controlled' experiments, in which 366 sick soldiers were treated by one of three surgeons assigned on rotation, one of whom used bloodletting while the other two did not. He found that the death rate was ten times higher in the soldiers treated with bloodletting.

The bloodletting practice was eventually abandoned for all but a few specific medical conditions, such as polycythaemia vera, a type of blood cancer in which the bone marrow makes too many red blood cells; and haemochromatosis, a genetic disorder that results in the body storing too much iron. Ingrained traditional practices are, however, hard to change, and the practice of bloodletting was still used and recommended well into the 20th century. In fact, a 1920 obstetrics textbook from Johns Hopkins University, discussing the treatment of eclampsia (shock associated with pregnancy that can result in death), suggested that if all else fails, doctors should try draining a pint of blood, which is probably the worst thing you could possibly do in that situation, as it further reduces the capacity of the body to deliver oxygen to the baby and to the mother's vital organs. A few years later, one of the fathers of modern medicine, Sir William Osler, in his 1923 edition of the widely used textbook *The Principles and Practice of Medicine*, recommended bloodletting as a treatment option for pneumonia.

A good illustration of the power of tradition and personally held beliefs over scientific evidence can be found in the reaction of doctors to the publication of scientific work refuting the practice of bloodletting. In the *American Journal of Medical Sciences* in 1836, one doctor wrote: 'Physicians are not prepared to discard therapies validated by both tradition and their own experience on account of someone else's numbers'. This telling quote is an opinion shared by many doctors today when faced with evidence that contradicts tradition and their own beliefs.

We're frequently confronted with similar reactions when we give lectures or write papers on the evidence against certain medical practices, such as drug treatments for back pain and arthroscopy for symptomatic osteoarthritis of the knee. This problem of doctors not understanding, not believing or preferring to ignore the scientific evidence and holding fast to their fixed beliefs is at the root of the harms stemming from medicine as it's practised today.

The legacy of medical harms from surgery

Surgeons and their predecessors have been around for as long as physicians. From thousands of years ago, there's evidence from diverse places such as Ancient Greece, North and South America, Africa, Polynesia and the Far East of trepanation: drilling a hole in the skull to release 'evil'. This practice is thought to have been developed independently by peoples in these various locations. And since then, surgeons have been cutting off limbs and operating on organs in the name of some very questionable theories.

It wasn't simply a matter of the surgery being ineffective, it very often resulted in death. Even the advent of anaesthesia, a boon to surgery, only made the surgery itself more tolerable for the patient – it didn't change the risks of the surgery. In one of the earliest amputations under anaesthesia, early in the 19th century, Robert Liston, a famous Scottish surgeon with a reputation for speed, performed a leg amputation that resulted in the deaths of three people: the patient, the assistant (whose two fingers were amputated in the process) and a spectator who had a heart attack watching it. In another amputation Liston completed in under three minutes, he inadvertently also cut off the patient's testicles.

As recently as the 20th century, doctors were removing various organs to treat psychiatric disease. Like bloodletting, this wasn't some crackpot idea but part of mainstream medicine. The two best documented cases were removing a woman's uterus (hysterectomy) and destroying part of the brain (lobotomy), but a more recent example is bone marrow transplantation for breast cancer.

Hysterectomy

For centuries, doctors thought the uterus could wander about the body, causing symptoms – even Hippocrates wrote of it. Indeed, 'hysteria' (which originates from the Greek word *hystera* meaning 'uterus'), was named to indicate that its symptoms (anxiety, shortness of breath, fainting, insomnia, irritability, nervousness and sexually forward behaviour) were attributable to a 'wandering' uterus. We probably don't need to point out that it was men who were making this diagnosis. The unlucky patients with hysteria were treated with hysterectomy. This procedure remains in common use today, although for different but sometimes still questionable reasons, such as endometriosis. It wasn't until 1952 that the American Psychiatric Association dropped the term 'hysteria'.

Lobotomy

As recently as the middle of the 20th century, doctors were performing frontal lobotomies that destroyed parts of the brain, sometimes by using an icepick inserted above the eyes, for poorly defined mental and behavioural problems, including depression, panic disorder, mania and schizophrenia. It worked, in terms of getting rid of the behavioural problems, but at the expense of a person's personality and intellect; some people died or committed suicide and others were left with severe brain injury.

The inventor of the procedure, Portuguese neurologist António

Egas Moniz, received a Nobel prize for Physiology or Medicine in 1949 for discovering its therapeutic value in certain psychoses. By 1951, almost 20 000 lobotomies had been performed in the United States and proportionally more in the United Kingdom, the majority on women. Like bloodletting before it, lobotomy is now a disparaged procedure, a symbol of medical barbarism but also an example of medical hubris.

From today's perspective, the types of treatments used in the past might look like the complete opposite of what was needed: bloodletting to treat people suffering blood loss from wounds; tying off the carotid artery, which supplies blood to the brain, for strokes due to a lack of blood to the brain; deliberately leaving material in surgical wounds to 'encourage the generation of pus'. It was a credit to the resilience and healing powers of the body that many patients survived these treatments. It also highlights an important problem: because some patients survived and recovered, the doctors attributed the recovery to their treatment. This logical fallacy of *post hoc ergo propter hoc* (Latin for 'after this, therefore because of this') is a strong reason why ineffective treatments persist.

Bone marrow transplantation for breast cancer

This procedure from more recent times involved transplanting bone marrow cells previously harvested from breast cancer patients (technically a 'rescue' or 'self-transplant') in order to allow the delivery of very high (otherwise fatal) doses of chemotherapy. The thinking was that if some chemotherapy was good, more was better (as for some blood cancers). Of course, such treatment was *potentially* very dangerous – lots of harms can occur with bone marrow transplant, let alone high-dose chemotherapy – but also *potentially* very helpful.

This would normally be an ideal situation for a comparative or 'controlled' clinical trial, a study that compares a group of patients who receive the treatment to a group who don't receive the treatment – the best way to test if treatments really work. But instead of any sort of controlled trial, it was simply *assumed* to be beneficial based on observing that some patients got better. We call this *observational* evidence, and it usually doesn't allow us to conclude that patients got better *because of* the treatment. This rather startling revelation, that the practice was accepted simply because some patients got better, sounds flippant but is true: there was no high-quality (in a scientific sense) comparative evidence that this rather radical treatment was better than standard treatment or that it was helping people and not harming them.

By the 1990s the practice of bone marrow rescue had really taken off in some settings, particularly in the US, and health insurers were sued for millions if they didn't cover this (very expensive) treatment. This was in part due to the publication of highly positive, but totally fraudulent, purported comparative studies conducted by cancer specialist Dr Werner Bezwoda in South Africa, but it was also driven by the beliefs of the doctors performing the procedure.

At the end of the 1990s, the high-quality evidence from legitimate comparative trials had finally been generated and the jury was in: it didn't work. The practice was stopped, but not before many women with breast cancer had undergone bone marrow transplantation with high-dose chemotherapy and its attendant dangers, including infection, severe mouth ulcers (mucositis), low blood counts leading to anaemia and low platelet counts leading to bleeding, for absolutely no benefit. Not only that, but many women died as a direct result of the treatment. It's estimated that about 30 000 women worldwide underwent this procedure and 1–3 per cent of them died as a result.

It's worth noting that the clinical trials took a lot longer than usual to complete. The results of the earlier studies were so positive that women were reluctant to be part of a trial where they had a fifty-fifty chance of *not* receiving the bone marrow transplant. They wanted the new treatment based upon what they were led to believe were highly promising results at the time.

The big leap

Sometimes treatments are introduced based on scientific evidence, but that evidence may not be directly applicable to humans – that is, it might be laboratory evidence or evidence from animal experiments. Again, the doctors jump to the conclusion that it *probably* works before getting the *real* evidence from real patients. In the 1990s, for example, antioxidant vitamins A and E were recommended by doctors based on evidence that oxidation in cells in the lab is a bad thing. While this may be true, it's a big leap to then say that an antioxidant will help people. 'People' are an unbelievably complex combination of lots of cells that don't live in a lab. By focusing only on the potential benefit, the doctors overlooked important questions. What other effects might these antioxidants have? Are they toxic at high doses? What are the unintended consequences? *After* antioxidant supplements were promoted and widely used, a summary of the evidence of their effectiveness in reducing mortality, based upon 67 trials involving more than 200 000 participants, concluded that there were more deaths among people who took the vitamins than those who didn't, and they were benefiting no one.

Sometimes, rather than being *completely* ineffective, some treatments *are* effective only for a particular patient group but are then somehow used much more widely to treat people outside that group. For example, while there may be a role for tonsillectomy in some cases, at one stage it was being performed on the majority of children in many regions of the world (see chapter 3).

Treating people who aren't sick: thalidomide

There are numerous examples of drugs being given to completely healthy people and causing significant harm – thalidomide is one such tragic example. Thalidomide was sold to the world as the 'wonder drug' for morning sickness from the mid-1950s to the early 1960s. The drug was developed by the West German pharmaceutical company Chemie Grünenthal and was sold over the counter, no prescription needed. Soon it was produced and sold by other pharmaceutical companies under licence to Grünenthal. It was marketed for pregnant women in 46 countries, including Australia, New Zealand, the United Kingdom and Canada, and prescribed to hundreds of thousands of women. It was never tested on pregnant animals, let alone humans, and it was falsely and heavily promoted as completely safe in pregnancy.

Incidentally, it was never marketed in the United States because Frances Kelsey, a Canadian–American pharmacologist and physician who reviewed the drug for the US Food and Drug Administration (FDA) had concerns about the lack of evidence regarding its safety. John F Kennedy later made her only the second woman to receive the prestigious President's Award for Distinguished Federal Civilian Service.

Thalidomide caused one of the biggest medical disasters in history – birth defects in an estimated 20 000 babies, and another 80 000 who died in the womb or were stillborn. The tragedy led to a worldwide overhaul in the regulation of medicines.

While thalidomide was withdrawn from the market in 1961 in Australia and many other countries, it was reintroduced in 2001 to treat rare diseases such as leprosy and some bone marrow cancers. New generations of 'thalidomiders' are being born in places such as Brazil and Argentina, despite inserts, and the pill bottles themselves, warning of the risks to pregnant women and strict regulations for prescribing the drug to women. In areas with a high prevalence of leprosy, there's also widespread sharing of medication and poor health education. The warning label, an image of a pregnant woman with a cross through it, has been misinterpreted, so the pills are also sold as a contraceptive.

Treating the numbers, not the disease: rosiglitazone

In diabetes, blood sugar levels have been the measure of treatment success or failure for a long time. But the problem with relying on the numbers alone was shown when some new diabetes drugs were released onto the market in 1999 after studies showed they could lower blood sugar levels. One of these drugs, rosiglitazone, was later thought to increase the risk of heart attack and sudden death compared to other diabetes drugs and placebos (pills with no drug included). To be clear: the blood sugars *were* lower in people using rosiglitazone, but they were also more likely to die. Rather than withdraw the drug, the US FDA initially elected to put a warning on the box and only withdrew the drug later when the evidence became even clearer. The drug was on the market for more than ten years, with worldwide sales peaking at about US$3 billion per year.

In the wash-up, an FDA advisory committee noted that rosiglitazone, 'a new "wonder drug", approved prematurely and for the wrong reasons by a weakened and underfunded government agency subjected to pressure from industry, had caused undue harm to patients'. The chair of the committee also noted: 'we urgently need to change the regulatory pathway for drugs for the treatment of type 2 diabetes to make clinical outcomes, not surrogates, the primary end points'. New diabetes drugs now need be evaluated in trials with cardiovascular outcomes to ensure they do not cause harm before they can be approved by the FDA.

The role of the pharmaceutical companies in hiding unfavourable study results, intimidating doctors who were critical of the drug, and downplaying the safety risks when promoting the drug, has been discussed at length elsewhere. While they have been rightly blamed for the rosiglitazone disaster, we are more interested here in the role of the doctors.

In one regard, the doctors were merely following the evidence they had been given, and recommendations from the FDA. At the end of the day, however, it is the doctor's signature on the prescription, so they bear the responsibility of making sure the drug is safe and effective. Doctors were also involved in research into the drug, some of which was withheld from publication, and many doctors were paid by the manufacturers. Conflicted doctors even lobbied regulators to keep the drug on the market and sat on the committees that decided that the drug should not be withdrawn. It is easy to paint the drug companies and government regulators as the bad guys, and the doctors as the heroes, but it is often not the case. Drug companies take an 'oath' to maximise profit for shareholders, but it is the doctors who are supposed to 'do no harm'; their oath is to the patients.

Solving a non-existent issue: the opioid epidemic

Perhaps the strongest current example of how our best intentions have led to massive harm is the opioid epidemic. It has been most prominent in the United States, but has also affected Canada, Australia and Europe. It's also ravaging the developing world, including India, Africa and the Middle East, in what the United Nations has dubbed the 'other opioid crisis', as it has generated far less publicity.

This tragedy is an 'iatrogenic' epidemic, meaning it was caused by doctors and the medical system. It has been called the biggest mistake ever made in the history of modern medical pain management. These drugs were given with the best intention – to relieve pain – but the estimates of how effective they were, as well as their possible harms, were way off.

In the early 1990s, there was widespread concern that there was an epidemic of untreated acute pain in American hospitals. Studies were showing that emergency department nurses and others were significantly underestimating patients' pain compared to patient self-report. By the middle of the decade, the American Pain Society had floated the idea that pain should be the fifth 'vital sign', essential information to be collected at every encounter with a patient, alongside the other vital signs of pulse rate, blood pressure, temperature and respiration (breathing) rate.

This concept caught on rapidly, and the rating of a patient's pain on a numerical scale became mandatory. At the same time, it became obligatory to treat the pain. No large studies were ever performed to determine whether the assessment of a person's pain on a routine basis either improved pain assessment or significantly reduced patients' pain levels. While there were some early concerns about whether there was really a need to screen *all* patients for the presence of pain and whether this might lead to overuse of opioids, others made it a human rights issue. There was even a Global Day Against Pain campaign held in 2004 to promote pain relief as a human right.

The measurement of pain became one of the 'quality of care' indicators used in the accreditation of hospitals, and rather than treating pain on an as-needed basis, treatment algorithms were developed to ensure pain would be 'eliminated'.

While it was well intentioned, making pain a vital sign has had profound unintended consequences. Although doctors had traditionally been very cautious in their use of opioid analgesia (pain relief) for people with chronic non-cancer pain due to concerns about tolerance, dependence and addiction, the number of prescriptions for opioids in the United States started to increase on an annual basis from the early 1990s, and in the late 1990s it accelerated. Doctors were falsely reassured by weak evidence and industry claims that addiction rates were very low.

In 1995 a new sustained-release longer-acting opioid called oxycodone (marketed as OxyContin) was approved by the US FDA for treating pain. The approved labelling stated that addiction from the drug was 'very rare' and the delayed absorption reduced the potential for abuse. These unsubstantiated claims weren't removed until 2001. In fact, the maker of the drug, Purdue Pharma, ensured that these claims were greatly reinforced, using paid expert doctors to speak on the subject.

By 2012, 255 million prescriptions for opioids were being filled annually by US retail pharmacies, which equates to 81.3 prescriptions per 100 people. According to the US National Institute on Drug Abuse, data from 2018 indicated that more than 128 Americans were dying every day after overdosing on opioids, including prescription opioids, heroin and synthetic opioids such as fentanyl (also a prescribed medicine). According to the US Centers for Disease Control and Prevention, more than 42 000 Americans died from opioid overdose in 2016, the last year for which data are available. About 2 million people are estimated to suffer from substance abuse disorders related to prescription opioids, while another half a million suffer from heroin addiction – there's overlap in the use of these drugs.

About a quarter of patients prescribed opioids for chronic pain misuse them. This means they might take them in a way other than prescribed, including in a higher dose, or they might take them to get high. About one in ten people prescribed opioids develop an opioid addiction, and about 80 per cent of people who use heroin first misused prescription opioids. There's also no sign that this public health tragedy in the United States (or elsewhere) is abating – opioid overdoses continue to increase in most US states by more than 30 per cent annually and over 50 per cent in some large cities. In fact, while the US comprises just under 5 per cent of the world's population, it uses more than 80 per cent of the world's supply of opioids.

But this doesn't mean other countries are immune. Australia saw a 15-fold increase in opioid dispensing between 1992 and 2012, and, as in the US, the increase has been greatest in regional and rural areas. This has been accompanied by an increase in prescription opioid deaths which now account for about a quarter of all drug-related deaths, about a third of which are due to fentanyl (which is 100 times stronger than morphine). While in the 1990s, heroin deaths were 2.5 times more common than prescription opioid deaths, the reverse is now true.

Over the years, Purdue Pharma has settled numerous US federal and state charges for millions of dollars. It has pleaded guilty to deceptively claiming that OxyContin is less addictive, less subject to misuse and less likely to cause dependence than other pain medicines; promoting off-label use of the drug; and deceptive marketing.

In an effort to increase revenue after it had declined following a reformulation of the drug to make it more difficult to misuse, and with clear knowledge of its detrimental effects including many preventable opioid-related deaths, the company focused on marketing the drug to high-prescribing doctors. These doctors make up less than 7 per cent of all prescribers but prescribe more opioids than the other 93 per cent of doctors combined. The company provided kickbacks to the highest prescribers (almost US$500 000 in one case) as well as to pharmacies willing to fill prescriptions other pharmacies declined to fill, and also conspired with an electronic health records company to create alerts suggesting OxyContin in medical software.

The latest settlement, in October 2020, resulted in resolution of all current US federal criminal and civic charges against both Purdue Pharma and its owners, the Sackler family, after they were allowed to enter plea agreements. Only three company executives have ever been fined, while no member of the Sackler family has ever confessed to doing anything wrong. The extraordinary role of the Sackler family in the promotion of opioids, including callous marketing to increase sales and minimisation of the harms, has nevertheless been the subject of many exposés, including two in the *New Yorker*. A 2021 perspective piece by Corey Davis in the *New England Journal of Medicine* has asked why Purdue Pharma and the Sackler family have not been served the justice they deserve for their illegal drug activities.

Meanwhile, in the developing world there has been mass abuse of the less potent opioid drug tramadol, originally developed by Grünenthal (the same pharmaceutical company that originally made thalidomide). Advocates have claimed that this is a less addictive opioid, yet dependence on the drug and misuse for its stimulant effects is rife. In Egypt, for example, of all people treated in state addiction facilities, 70 per cent are addicted to tramadol; while in Nigeria, tramadol misuse affects just over half the population, and more than 90 per cent obtain it without a prescription. It's claimed that this has occurred due to loopholes in regulation that have accompanied an underestimate of the drug's dangers. A 2019 *Los Angeles Times* investigative report focusing on tramadol suggests that Grünenthal has campaigned to keep the drug unregulated, claiming that the problem lies with illicit counterfeit pills, and that putting tighter controls in place would make it difficult for patients with pain to access the drug.

So how did this all happen? Once pain was mandated as a vital sign, doctors were expected to ask patients if they had any pain. If any pain was reported, doctors were expected to prescribe treatment to either reduce the pain or eliminate it completely. And they conditioned patients to expect that this would occur. At the same time, however, most clinicians lacked adequate knowledge about how to assess and manage pain. They didn't recognise that for many people, prescribing opioids wasn't the correct response. Yet prescribing opioids, and in high and escalating doses, became the mantra to alleviate pain and suffering. They had forgotten about 'first, do no harm'.

As doctors, we've seen the effects in our day-to-day practices of this expectation that all pain must be eliminated. We regularly see patients who were prescribed opioids for an acute episode of pain, such as an injury, and it simply gets continued. After a short time, the patient finds they are irritable, in more pain, sometimes have nausea, and have difficulty sleeping if they stop taking the drug, so their doctor prescribes more, not realising that the symptoms are not from the original injury, but from the opioids themselves. Paradoxically, opioids are the cause and the cure for the problem of opioids, so they keep getting prescribed. We can attest to how difficult it is to explain this to patients and to get them off the drugs, especially compared to the relative simplicity of writing another prescription.

Perhaps the biggest twist in this tale of opioids is that the drugs aren't all that effective in the first place for non-cancer pain. They often don't relieve pain any more than other (non-opioid) drugs and they nearly all have terrible effects on people, both physically (drowsiness and constipation are very common) and psychologically.

Seeing this problem in patients discharged after surgery, we conducted a blinded scientific study (a randomised controlled trial) comparing the usual, strong opioid (OxyContin) prescribed to patients at discharge from hospital following surgery, to a much milder type of opioid-plus-paracetamol drug, then available over the counter. We gave patients either the OxyContin or the milder drug, and both were identically packaged, so they didn't know which one they were taking. The study showed no difference in the levels of pain in the days and weeks following discharge, and no difference in the numbers of pills taken (patients were allowed to adjust the dose according to their pain). In fact, the only difference between these two groups of patients was that the rate of complications was much higher in the patients who took the stronger drug. While this has changed our own prescribing patterns, changing practice on a larger scale is much more difficult.

There's much less evidence than we thought for the superiority of strong opioids over less harmful drugs, and researchers are only now doing the studies that should have been completed decades ago, such as comparing opioids to placebo drugs. Why had nobody done these studies before? Because we just assumed that the stronger the opioid, the better it must be at relieving pain.

Could medicinal cannabis be the answer?

Most probably not. We've all seen news articles about people who swear by it, as do many doctors. But we can't assume effectiveness just because we see some people get better or because we *want* it to work; we have to rely on good science. And the most reputable evidence about medicinal cannabis for just about anything (chronic cancer or non-cancer pain, nausea, dementia, arthritis, spasms) indicates that it's either not very effective or not effective at all.

A study published in the *British Medical Journal* summarising all the available evidence for medical cannabis for both chronic non-cancer and cancer-related pain, with follow-up of at least a month, found that there was only a small chance of improving pain, and even then, the improvement itself was small. These results appeared similar irrespective of whether the pain was due to cancer or other causes.

At best only one in ten study participants experienced any improvement in pain compared with taking a placebo. On average their pain was only about 0.5 out of ten better. Even smaller benefits were seen for physical functioning and sleep quality. In addition, compared with taking a placebo, about one in ten participants experienced dizziness, while a lower number (2–5 per cent) also experienced nausea, vomiting, drowsiness, impaired attention and/or transient impairment in thinking. These findings were also in keeping with a review informing the 2019 UK guidance for medical cannabis, which concluded that the average effect on pain was negligible.

Why do we keep getting it so wrong?

All the examples we have outlined in this chapter have caused or are continuing to cause harm. They were all well intentioned, but they show us how good intentions and personal experience alone are an inadequate basis for practising medicine. Our patients deserve and should expect more – our intentions and actions need to be supported by science.

A core problem, and the reason behind much of the excess in health care, lies in the mismatch between *perceptions* of the benefits and harms of medical care and their *true* effects. There's considerable evidence that doctors' estimates of the benefits of what they do aren't accurate, they're *overestimated*; while at the same time their estimates of the harms coming from what they do are also wrong – they're *underestimated*.

This problem isn't confined to doctors. Patients do the same thing. A 2015 review of studies on this topic found that about two-thirds of patients overestimate the benefits they will receive from treatments and around two-thirds also underestimate the harms. In fact, these faulty estimates of the benefits and harms of health care are prevalent in the community, and likely stem from the way they're portrayed by both doctors and others: the benefits are overstated while the harms are under-reported.

Let's suppose, for example, that you're a 60-year-old man with knee pain and you search Dr Google for information on knee arthroscopy to see whether it's worth considering. Nearly all the sites you come across will paint a rosy picture of the procedure, while only about 15 per cent will explain that it actually provides no worthwhile benefits. Most sites will give some information about the potential risks, but far fewer will provide explicit information about their likelihood, and this will vary widely depending on the site.

We know this because in 2017 we studied these sites. About half of them were websites based in Australia, while most of the remainder were based in the United States. The owners of the websites varied – and included consumer information companies and organisations, government, health insurers, professional societies, hospitals and orthopaedic surgeons – and none mentioned the availability of guidelines or their recommendations. Our findings concur with many similar studies.

The media also often provide unbalanced information in their desire to capture the readers' attention. Harms from medicine are hardly reported, and instead there is a constant flow of good-news stories and breakthroughs that often overstate the benefits. Even things that have been shown to provide no significant benefit are heralded as life-saving breakthroughs. The use of robots in surgery, for example, is often hyped in the media. Hospitals are spending millions buying these robots, despite little evidence that their use improves patient outcomes compared to traditional, non-robotic surgery. This is just as true for prostatectomy and hysterectomy as for removing gall bladders or doing knee replacements. In fact, a recent review suggests that in some areas they may be making things worse.

To test whether newer is always better, researchers who reviewed new hip and knee replacement devices introduced in Australia over a five-year period found that nearly 30 per cent of them performed worse than the established replacements, and that none of the new devices performed better.

'Breakthrough' cancer drugs are no different. Their benefits are often wildly overstated in the media, although of course there are exceptions that *are* genuine breakthrough drugs, such as immunotherapy with checkpoint inhibitors for several cancers including melanoma, and some targeted therapies for specific cancers. In a study of newly approved cancer drugs in the United

States, however, it was noted that, at the time of approval, most had no evidence of improving quality of life or survival times. Years later, most of them had still shown no clinical benefit to survival. Cancer drugs are often initially approved for use and reimbursement based on their ability to shrink the size of a tumour or improve disease-free survival, rather than their effect on overall survival. The ability to make people live longer (*overall* survival) is arguably the outcome that's most important.

A review of 71 consecutive cancer drugs approved for 'solid' tumours (excluding blood cancers such as leukemia) between 2002 and 2012 showed that the median improvement in survival was 2.1 months – including hospitalisation, the time taken to give the drug, and the time spent unwell while taking the drug. The benefits are likely to be smaller in the real world, where (for example) discontinuation rates are higher due to the ill effects of having the treatment.

Why the rose-coloured glasses?

Why do we maintain this constantly positive view of medicine? We can think of at least six reasons:

1 *It's what we (doctors and patients, and their carers)* want *to believe*

Doctors want to believe that what they're doing is helping their patients. They're also more open to and accepting of evidence that supports their beliefs. The term for this is 'confirmation bias' – the tendency to seek out, interpret and recall information in a way that confirms our existing beliefs. And when we're faced with evidence contrary to our beliefs, our tendency is to find flaws in the evidence in order to dismiss it. This is the way our minds deal with the 'cognitive dissonance' created by incompatible or conflicting views.

2   There's uncertainty

Sometimes we just don't know the precise probabilities of risk and benefit because there's insufficient evidence. In times of uncertainty, our biases kick in and we *assume* effectiveness rather than wait for the evidence that establishes the truth. Uncertainty is often used as an excuse to treat rather than wait.

3   We don't understand the evidence

Sometimes the evidence is there, and the doctors have seen it and tried to be objective about evaluating it, but don't have the necessary scientific knowledge and skills to do so. This reflects the lack of training among doctors in clinical epidemiology (the basic science of clinical medicine) and statistics (see chapter 2). It's a common misconception that doctors are well trained in these scientific methods and critical appraisal, but this is very often not the case.

4   Miracle thinking

Even when we know the numbers, we distort the probabilities associated with success and failure, thinking that although the odds are stacked against us, we might get lucky. This is also called the lottery mentality. When we buy lottery tickets, we overestimate our chances of winning (*benefiting*) when the chances are actually very low (say, one in 1 million). But when it comes to our chances of losing (*being harmed*), we discount or dismiss altogether events that might be much more likely. For example, a one in 1000 chance of dying from surgery is often seen as highly unlikely.

5   We're too easily misled

As a result of not understanding the science, we're susceptible to unsupported claims. We're repeatedly and convincingly told that treatments work, by advertisers, company representatives, colleagues, friends and neighbours, and by news reports of great medical success. It can be hard to see through the rhetoric and marketing spin that accompanies new tests and treatments, often helped along by paid and sometimes 'coached' medical opinion leaders. This is why it's so important for doctors to understand the science and remain independent.

6   It's in our interests

Finally, deep down it's in everybody's interests for a treatment to work. Without having a treatment to offer, doctors can feel devalued and ineffective. Assuming an intervention works is what keeps people in jobs and businesses in profit; not just the doctors, but anybody supplying the health industry. It's also in the patient's and their family's interests to believe a treatment will be effective.

Medical care is also harming our planet

Too much medical care doesn't just harm individuals, it also has detrimental effects on the planet, which in turn results in further environment-related threats to our health. As we noted in the introduction, it has been estimated that about 7 per cent of Australia's total carbon footprint is due to health care. Half comes from hospitals and another 20 per cent from pharmaceuticals.

This is consistent with the fact that Australia has one of the highest per capita carbon emissions in the world. The comparable contribution to the national carbon footprint from health care in the United States has been estimated to be 10 per cent. Both are considerably more than the 4 per cent attributed to health care in the United Kingdom, which has been actively trying to reduce its healthcare-related carbon emissions since the UK Climate Change Act was passed in 2008. To support the National Health Service (NHS), public health and social care to create a sustainable, low-carbon health service, the Sustainable Development Unit (now called Greener NHS) was formed. As a result, the NHS has taken significant steps over the last decade towards reducing the impact of health care on climate and made a commitment to a 'net zero' NHS by 2040.

First, since 2008 the NHS has measured its carbon footprint and the progress made in reducing it. Some hospitals have switched to 100 per cent renewable electricity, including low-carbon heating and lighting; reduced their wastage, particularly from single-use plastics and paper; and switched to fleets of electric cars. There has also been a significant decline in use of metered-dose inhalers that deliver asthma medications and general anaesthetic gases such as desflurane, both of which have large detrimental environmental effects. In 2019–20, 754 UK general practices accessed the Green Impact for Health toolkit to make their practices more sustainable, while all health services in the United Kingdom must now have clear plans for how they will achieve this.

Hospitals consume vast amounts of energy in the form of heating, electricity and water, and the goods and services they deliver. They use a lot of non-recyclable plastics and also produce, and need to dispose of, vast amounts of medical waste. Life-cycle assessment is one method used to measure the whole environmental footprint of a product or service, from acquiring the raw materials, processing, manufacturing, distribution and transportation, right through to its use, including its reuse and maintenance, and recycling and waste management. This can determine the impacts on carbon dioxide emissions, water and pollution.

This approach has been used to measure the environmental impacts of opioids (from the poppy farm to the packaged drug), hysterectomies, anaesthetic drugs and common hospital pathology tests. These studies have all highlighted the environmental gains that could be made by considering the environmental impacts of health care and, importantly, the gains that could be made by reducing unnecessary care.

Doctors are still largely unaware of the environmental harms of too much medicine. Yet, as early proponents of incorporating broad environmental standards into hospital accreditation processes in Australia, Drs Forbes McGain and Grant Blashki, together with engineer Kevin Moon and nurse Fiona Armstrong, wrote in the *Medical Journal of Australia* fifteen years ago, 'if the principle underpinning the work of all health professionals is *"do no harm"*, addressing the harmful effects of the health care industry on the natural environment must become a priority'.

* * *

By underestimating the harms and overestimating the benefits of what they do, doctors are harming patients in record numbers, often without any chance of benefit. In doing so, they have violated the first principle of medicine, to 'first, do no harm'.

2

Science matters

Hippocratic Oath: I will respect the hard-won scientific gains
of those physicians in whose steps I walk, and gladly share such
knowledge as is mine with those who are to follow.

'There are in fact two things, science and opinion;
the former begets knowledge, the latter ignorance'
– attributed to Hippocrates

'Science is a beautiful gift to humanity;
we should not distort it'
– APJ Abdul Kalam, Indian scientist and former president

To 'respect the hard-won scientific gains' means *knowing* the
evidence (the science) behind any decision, and also *incorporating*
it appropriately into practice. Unfortunately, we see failures in both
respects: doctors who don't know the best evidence, and doctors
who are aware of the evidence but don't incorporate it into their
decision-making. One of the best contemporary examples of this
is handwashing.

A brief history of handwashing

The germ theory of disease, first attributed to an Italian physician
and poet, Girolamo Fracastoro (1478–1553), proposed that many
diseases are caused by bacteria or other microorganisms. This

theory was largely dismissed for several hundred years because of the lack of any scientific proof of the existence of microorganisms that could cause illness.

The medical community often rejects new knowledge when it conflicts with established opinions, sometimes ridiculing those who challenge their accepted beliefs. This reflex-like rejection of new knowledge because it contradicts entrenched norms, beliefs or paradigms, has been coined the 'Semmelweis reflex', after the Hungarian physician Ignaz Semmelweis (1818–65), whose observations and ideas were ridiculed and rejected by his contemporaries.

In 1847 Semmelweis discovered that fever after childbirth (puerperal fever), a common complication in new mothers that was often fatal, could be drastically reduced by the practice of washing hands with an antiseptic (chlorinated lime solution) before examining patients. Despite the astounding results (deaths following childbirth were reduced from more than 10 per cent to about 1 per cent), his observations conflicted with established opinions. At that time there was still no proof that microorganisms could cause disease, so there was no acceptable explanation for his findings. Some doctors were even offended at the suggestion that they should have to wash their hands!

Sadly, it wasn't until years after Semmelweis's death that Louis Pasteur, a French biologist, microbiologist and chemist (1822–95), confirmed the germ theory and the Hungarian received the credit and acceptance he was due. Building on the work of Semmelweis and Pasteur, Joseph Lister, a British surgeon (1827–1912), proved the link between the lack of cleanliness in hospitals and deaths after operations. In a similar way to Semmelweiss, he found that he could reduce deaths following limb amputation, from around 50 per cent to 15 per cent, by using an antiseptic (carbolic acid, now known as phenol) that kills microorganisms to sterilise surgical instruments and clean wounds.

So how are we doing now in reducing the risk of spreading germs based upon Semmelweis's observation from more than 150 years ago? Do doctors and other healthcare professionals routinely wash their hands or use disinfectant *before* seeing patients? According to the World Health Organization (WHO), at any one time, seven out of 100 patients in developed countries and ten out of 100 in developing countries will acquire at least one healthcare-associated infection. Many of these are preventable through proper hand-hygiene techniques on the part of medical professionals. Only the recent advent of regular *compulsory* hand-hygiene training for hospital accreditation over the last decade has improved rates of hand hygiene in hospitals.

Before the COVID-19 pandemic, the most recent data showed that 15 per cent of healthcare workers were still not complying with optimal hand-hygiene methods (and doctors remained the most noncompliant). The pandemic resulted in an improvement in hand-hygiene practices in hospitals, although these improvements may not be sustained over the longer term. An increased perception of personal risk, and therefore the perceived need to protect themselves and their family, has been suggested to explain at least some of the observed improvements. In addition to social distancing, masks and of course border closures, it is likely that good hand-hygiene practices have also contributed to reduced flu and cold rates in Australia and around the world during the COVID pandemic.

Respecting the science

Doctors are often quick to claim the scientific high ground when challenging practitioners outside mainstream medicine, but are not so quick to apply those standards to their own practice. For example, it's common for doctors to criticise alternative practitioners such as homeopaths, naturopaths and chiropractors because many of their treatments lack supporting evidence from rigorously conducted randomised controlled trials. Yet many of those same doctors are unaware that many of their own practices also lack such supporting evidence.

Although the public assume that doctors practice medicine based largely upon scientific principles, much of what they do – the tests they order and the treatments they prescribe – have either not been proven to work or are supported by only weak evidence. In fact, it has been estimated that less than half the treatments prescribed today are supported by adequate evidence. Much remains unstudied, and therefore much medical care is based upon the individual clinician's judgment, which we know to be highly variable, often arbitrary and frequently wrong. Those hard-won scientific gains are either yet to be made or are ignored.

One example was illustrated by a recent review of the evidence behind surgery for musculoskeletal pain, including low back pain, shoulder pain, neck pain and osteoarthritis. These are among the most common health complaints and the most common reasons people visit a doctor.

The review looked at all published studies of 14 of the most common surgical procedures performed in this field, including joint replacement, spinal fusion, carpal tunnel decompression and arthroscopic surgery. It only included the 6782 studies that randomised participants to either having the surgery or not having the surgery, because these types of studies best indicate whether having the procedure is better than not having it. The people who did not have the surgery usually had some form of non-surgical treatment, such as exercises, or placebo surgery (where an incision is made but the surgery is not actually performed).

Less than 1 per cent of all the randomised trials published (only 64) compared doing the surgery with not doing the surgery. Most of the trials simply compared different surgical techniques or devices. In other words, they didn't actually answer the question of whether surgery worked at all. This may seem surprising but was expected: most doctors believe the surgery they perform works, and are disinclined to perform a study that tests that assumption. Some surgeons even find such studies unethical, as it denies the surgery to half the patients. We feel that the opposite is true: surgical procedures should not be performed unless they have passed such tests. To perform surgery that isn't supported by good evidence is unethical.

Even more surprising, however, was that most of the studies comparing surgery to no surgery showed that doing the surgery wasn't better than not doing it. In fact, only nine of the 64 studies showed surgery to be the preferred treatment.

Even when the scientific evidence is available, many doctors don't accept it or act on it. A 2003 study from the United States examined how doctors manage 30 common conditions, such as type 2 diabetes, headache and asthma, and compared this to how doctors *should* manage these conditions based on high-quality scientific evidence. They found that the recommended care was adhered to (on average) just over half the time. So even when doctors know what works, they provide the correct care only about half the time. Breaking these results down a little further, the study found that just under half the patients did not receive the care they should have, while just over 10 per cent of patients received care that wasn't recommended and was potentially harmful.

And this isn't unique to the United States. A study from Australia looking at more than 35 000 healthcare encounters with over 7000 patients found that they received appropriate care in only 57 per cent of cases.

Practice change is slow

The general public should rightly presume that doctors and other clinicians would endeavour to incorporate new evidence into clinical practice as soon as it becomes available. But as we have seen, there are large gaps between what we know and what we do. Apart from the huge task of keeping up to date with new evidence, simply 'knowing' the evidence is only step one in a long path towards 'doing' or enacting the evidence. This usually takes years and often takes decades. Professor Paul Glasziou, an Australian general practitioner and expert in evidence-based medicine, calls the 'knowing' part 'awareness' and describes it as only the first step in getting evidence into practice. Evidence must also be accepted, applicable, available, and able to be carried out, acted upon, agreed and adhered to. Each one of these can be a considerable hurdle, which is why it has been estimated that it takes around 17 years for new research to make its way into usual practice. Bridging this 'know–do gap' is considered one of the most important challenges for public health in this century. But as we will see, bridging the know–do gap has been a problem for centuries.

Why practice change is *so* slow

About a fifth of all research studies are never even written up for publication and therefore remain hidden. In many cases this is because the results were 'negative', meaning they weren't what the researchers had expected or wanted. This leads to a problem called 'publication bias'. Positive findings are more likely to get published than negative ones.

Even when the research is written up and the article submitted to a journal, nearly half are never accepted for publication. Sometimes the research has been rejected from many different journals. Even when studies are published, many still have technical flaws (for example, including too few people, or not using the right research methods to answer the question), so that their results are not reliable. And some studies aren't easily found because the central library that indexes them does not use the right words or terms to categorise them or may not list that particular journal at all.

Even after successfully navigating all these hurdles, it takes another six to 13 years for the results of published studies to be summarised or synthesised into reviews or recommendations for practice, and then *another* nine years for these to be taken up or incorporated into practice.

You might find it difficult to believe it really takes this long. But even when studies find that a new treatment or a new way of doing things is *vastly better* than the old one, it can take many years before this is translated into benefits to patients. A study published in 2000 highlights this problem. It estimated the proportion of people who were currently benefiting from landmark research findings published between 1968 and 1993. A pivotal trial published in 1968, for example, demonstrated the unequivocal benefits of flu vaccination for those at risk (such as older people), but in 2000 only 55 per cent of those at risk were receiving the flu vaccine. Similarly, only 20 per cent of people with diabetes were receiving routine foot care, although it was established to be beneficial in 1993. And only 20 per cent of heart attack patients were getting clot-busting drugs, despite a 1971 study showing them to be effective.

Why are we doing so badly? Why aren't we respecting the hard-won gains of science? Firstly, it's easy to distrust or disbelieve, and then dismiss, something you don't understand. Without a good understanding of the scientific method and therefore the reasons why a study might be more likely to be telling us the truth than a different study or than our own experience, it's easy to dismiss the research and go back to the comfort of tradition and your own experience. It's easier to continue to do what you've always done, and what everyone else is doing.

The teaching of scientific principles, including critical appraisal and problem-solving, receives much less emphasis than it should in medicine. Some doctors seek out and learn this for themselves, but most don't. Traditionally, the practice of clinical medicine has been taught by observing and imitating others, much like an apprenticeship. While this is essential for learning skills such as taking a history, performing a physical examination, taking blood or putting in an IV line, learning to critically question what we're doing and why has been given less emphasis. With today's ready availability of information there's less need for medical students to learn long lists of possible diagnoses for a given complaint or exact doses of medications. But it has become much more crucial that they can differentiate good-quality from poor-quality information. Seeking and appraising relevant new information as it becomes available should be a lifelong practice.

An understanding and respect for the science is crucial for doctors to keep up with the latest evidence and determine whether or not clinical practice should change. Yet teaching and reinforcing these skills is often missing from medical education, and in many specialties of medicine it is given scant, if any, attention. While it's a standard part of training for many physician specialties such as oncology, which has a rich history of science-based practice, other areas of medicine lag well behind. Critical appraisal skills (including knowledge of study design, statistics and other research methods) are *fundamental* to good medical care across all branches of medicine.

Despite recognition of this problem, and some improvements in medical training, many doctors today still don't have the skills to evaluate a research paper in a detailed and analytical way. It sounds absurd, but many would be unable to identify fatal flaws that would render the results of a study untrustworthy. They don't know how to determine which of two studies with conflicting results might be the more valid, and therefore more likely to be true. Even when the best available evidence is synthesised into guidelines or explicit recommendations for practice, doctors may have neither the motivation nor the skills to determine if this should prompt a change in their practice. In fact, it has been estimated that only one-third or less of guidelines are routinely followed in clinical practice. While there are many barriers to following guidelines (one study identified a total of 293 separate barriers), many barriers relate to doctors' knowledge, attitudes and ingrained beliefs about entrenched practices.

Ingrained beliefs are hard to shift

If you've been doing something one way for your whole career and someone tells you it doesn't work, your first thought is that they're wrong. And when we start to seek out the evidence, we tend to look for and are more likely to believe any that supports our previously held belief. This is the 'confirmation bias' we mentioned earlier, and it's a big problem in getting people to accept change.

Change is hard in any profession because professions are social groups. Nobody wants to stand out, partly because if you buck the trends you may be in trouble when it comes to defending your decisions against peers or in court or in medical meetings; unfortunately, it's simply easier to do what everyone else is doing. This is why, despite massive amounts of scientific evidence being published and released all over the world on a daily basis, practice change remains a social phenomenon – it occurs gradually, by direct human interaction.

Medical practices tend to be similar among doctors in the same social circle. It's very common, for example, for doctors at one hospital to all treat a condition a particular way, while all the doctors at another hospital will use a different treatment for the same condition. This is usually due to a lack of communication, or social interaction between doctors from different hospitals.

There are also, of course, financial reasons why we may not want to change, particularly if the change involves abandoning our major source of income. It's easy to understand that doctors who make much of their living inserting cardiac stents, for example, might not be inclined to agree with studies that show that stenting is no better than cheaper and safer treatments. They may focus on the flaws in the studies, highlight differences between patients in the study and their own patients, and even denigrate the skills of the doctors doing the stents in the study or criticise the types of stents used. The problems of financial incentives in medicine are discussed in more detail in chapter 7.

Sometimes doctors don't accept the science because they're just being human. Just as it's human nature to believe our own experience over the word of someone we've never met (like the author of a research study), it's also human nature to see cause and effect where only correlation exists. Evolutionarily, our brains were taught to jump to conclusions, to make a best guess and go with it when seeking causal explanations for the events we witness. This shortcut in thinking was an evolutionary advantage, for example if someone fell ill after eating a particular type of berry – we would *assume* that the berries were poisonous and no longer eat them. The assumption may or may not be true, but we lose little by making it.

These very human shortcuts in thinking weren't always helpful, however. For example, if someone killed a goat one day and the drought broke the next day, goat sacrifice might become the cure for any future droughts. This kind of magical thinking is not only the origin of many superstitions, but has also given rise to many traditional medical treatments. Until recently, 'cleaning out' the knee by performing keyhole surgery in people with arthritic knees was commonplace, based only on the perception that people felt better afterwards. It wasn't until many years after the treatment had become commonplace that high-quality studies comparing a washout to not performing a washout showed the treatment to be ineffective.

This shortcut we make is the logical fallacy called *post hoc ergo propter hoc* (it follows therefore it's because of) – and humans are hardwired to fall for it every time. We have to make a conscious and concerted effort to think through the logic of any given situation to avoid falling for the logical fallacy. What kept doctors in the bloodletting business for so long, is that some patients got better afterwards, therefore the doctors concluded they got better *because of* the treatment.

When this occurs, doctors are no different from the healers of the ancient times who used magic to heal their patients. The use of placebo treatments, along with manipulation of the clinical setting (adjusting patient expectations, for example), provides the same illusion of effectiveness.

Why science is the preferred way of knowing

There are scientific ways to test whether the patient got better *because* of a treatment or whether it was due to something else or if they would have recovered anyway. The best way to test whether a patient gets better *because* of the treatment is to perform a 'controlled' trial. This means assembling a group of similar patients with the same condition and treating one group with the treatment and another group, called the 'control' group, with a different treatment, or sometimes not treating them at all. With one group getting the treatment and the other group not getting the treatment, you can see how any difference in the recovery between the two groups might then be *fairly* attributed to the treatment.

One of the first 'controlled' trials in medicine was conducted in 1747 by a naval surgeon, James Lind (1716–94). He discovered that oranges and lemons given to one group of sailors with 'distemper at sea' stopped them dying, while observing that those not given the citrus fruit died. We now know that the 'distemper' was the disease scurvy, which is caused by a deficiency in vitamin C.

The idea of doing simple scientific comparative tests is easy to understand, but it was only in recent decades that it became routine and widely practised. And while it's now the gold standard for the introduction of new medications, many older, traditional treatments, such as the knee washout mentioned above, were 'grandfathered' in and never subjected to such tests. In fact, it's still not routine for newer surgical techniques, and it's rarely applied to determine the value of having a pathology test (e.g. blood, urine) or imaging scan (e.g. X-ray, CT or MRI).

The contemporary way of practising medicine is called 'evidence-based' medicine and is the integration of clinical experience and patient values *with* the best evidence to help individual patients make the best decisions about their health care. It's not all that different from 'traditional' medicine except that it requires a greater respect for the science. Simply relying on clinical experience and trust in tradition is no longer good enough. Reliance upon clinical experience has often led us astray and harmed people. New treatments that seem to be 'miraculous' when first used are often shown to be anything but miraculous upon more rigorous scientific testing.

By now you would have thought that people would be more sceptical of treatments that seem too good to be true. But patients around the world are continuing to be harmed (or at the very least not receiving benefit), from treatments proven to be ineffective.

In the 'hierarchy' of evidence, *experimental* evidence (controlled trials) always trumps *observational* evidence, which is simply a description of what happens when a group of patients are given a particular treatment as part of their usual care. Even among controlled trials, some are more trustworthy than others. It depends on how they use scientific tools such as 'randomisation', which means that patients have an equal chance of receiving one treatment or another because they are assigned a treatment at random. To make things even more objective, the highest-quality randomised controlled trials also blind the trial participants, their doctors and anyone else associated with the trial. This means that neither the participant nor anyone else knows which treatment the participant received, thus providing an even fairer test of the treatment. For example, blinding of all trial personnel in a drug trial can be achieved by using a placebo pill that is identical to the real thing except it doesn't contain the drug. Of course, *someone* needs to know who got what; but they keep the code secret, don't interact with anyone else involved in the trial, and the code is only broken after the results are analysed. Often, as the way a treatment is studied becomes more trustworthy, the benefits seem to shrink, sometimes until they disappear altogether.

The vertebroplasty affair

Severely painful fractures in the back, a condition that mostly affects older adults with osteoporosis (fragile bones), are common – there are about 700 000 new cases annually in the United States alone. In Australia there were estimated to be more than 25 500 in 2012 and this is expected to rise to over 35 000 by 2022.

They generally heal within a few weeks or months but until that time they may cause severe pain and disability. Vertebroplasty, a treatment that involves the injection of a type of acrylic cement into fractures in the spine (vertebral bodies), is a treatment that was first introduced in the late 1980s. It can be performed by various types of doctors, such as radiologists or surgeons. Early observations of people who had the procedure, published over the next 15 years, indicated that it quickly and dramatically improved pain. On average, across 30 *observational* studies, the pain improved from a score of about eight out of ten (where 0 indicates no pain and 10 very severe pain) to about a two and a half, and serious complications were reported in less than 1 per cent of patients. The treatment was widely hailed as a miracle – in June 2003, the London *Telegraph* reported it as an example of the 'Lazarus effect', enabling the bed-bound to walk again, and it rapidly became the standard of care.

The first *experimental* studies weren't performed until 2003 and 2006. In these controlled trials, all patients were offered the vertebroplasty, and those who declined became the control or comparison group. In the 2003 study, patients who received the vertebroplasty had significantly less pain straight after the procedure compared with those who declined it, but by six weeks, pain levels were similar in both groups. In the 2006 study, patients who had received vertebroplasty also did better and had less pain immediately after the procedure, but the patients in the treated group had much higher levels of pain to begin with. This seems to make sense when you consider that people who agreed to have a vertebroplasty might have been more desperate for pain relief than people who refused the treatment. If, however, you have higher pain levels to begin with, there's also more room for improvement, and so the comparison isn't a fair one. In this case, it's likely to have overestimated the value of the treatment. Because these studies didn't *randomly* allocate people to one treatment or the other, it's likely that the researchers were comparing apples with oranges: the people in the two treatment groups were different from each other in more ways than just the treatment they received.

The first randomised controlled trial of vertebroplasty, which wasn't conducted until 2007, only included a small number of people. It also found that those who received the vertebroplasty experienced greater pain relief immediately after the procedure, but this time, after two weeks, the levels of pain were the same in both groups. Like the previous studies, everyone involved in the trial, including the patients and the investigators, knew which treatments had been received – they weren't 'blinded'. This means that the benefits of treatment in the people who had the vertebroplasty could have been enhanced by an expectation that it was going to work, while the people in the control group, knowing they weren't receiving vertebroplasty, might have expected not to improve. The benefits of having the vertebroplasty could also have been enhanced by a staff member treating the patient being an enthusiastic advocate of the treatment.

The first two *randomised blinded* trials of vertebroplasty weren't published until 2009, more than 20 years after vertebroplasty had been introduced into practice. We should declare that Rachelle was the principal investigator on one of these trials. Unlike the previous trials, the comparison groups in both trials received a placebo procedure. This means that they were treated in exactly the same way as those in the vertebroplasty group, except they didn't have the vertebroplasty. They received medication to make them sleepy, an injection of local anaesthetic and a needle inserted into their back – everything, that is, except having the cement injected.

Because the participants in these trials were all blinded, any differences between the vertebroplasty and placebo groups can be attributed to the true effect of the vertebroplasty and not to other factors, such as how they were expecting to feel. Both trials also blinded the investigators, reducing the chance that they would somehow treat the two groups differently. The only people who weren't blinded were the ones doing the procedure, and they were under strict instructions to treat all trial participants in exactly the same way.

The results of these two trials were almost identical. In both, those who had received the placebo and those who had received the vertebroplasty improved by about the same amount. The vertebroplasty saga was chronicled in an excellent 2010 editorial written by Dr Eugene Carragee, an orthopaedic surgeon and editor of the *Spine Journal*. He titled it 'The vertebroplasty affair: the mysterious case of the disappearing effect size'.

Many people praised these two trials for finally establishing the truth about a treatment that had been introduced into practice before proper evaluation. Proponents of the procedure, however, greeted the study findings with disbelief (and worse). Because the results seemed to contradict what they had observed in practice, they attempted to discredit the trials. Predictably, they suggested that the wrong patients were studied – for example, their pain wasn't severe enough or they'd had the pain for too long – or the treatment wasn't given in the right way.

Further adding to the confusion, some professional groups, such as the American Academy of Orthopaedic Surgeons (AAOS) released strong recommendations *against* the use of vertebroplasty, while others, such as the UK National Institute for Health and Care Excellence (NICE), recommended *for* its use, stating that while the results of the two placebo-controlled trials raised questions about the effectiveness of vertebroplasty, they were convinced by clinical experience that seemed to show that the procedure worked. This is the exact opposite of how science should be understood: they are choosing to believe the *observational* evidence (including their own experience) over high-quality *experimental* studies that offer a more objective measure of the true effectiveness of the procedure. They're saying that they don't believe the high-quality evidence because it conflicts with their beliefs, the exact problem that an understanding of science is meant to address.

Three more placebo-controlled trials investigating this question have now been completed. The results of two of these trials were exactly the same as the previous trials and showed no benefit from vertebroplasty. The third trial claimed there were some limited benefits, but whether these were clinically relevant is debatable. Combining information from all of the trials gives convincing evidence that vertebroplasty is not beneficial.

Hundreds of thousands of patients have now received vertebroplasty. In many parts of the world, the practice still continues today, despite the weight of evidence against it. Not only that, many harms have also been reported, including infections, rib and further vertebral fractures, cement fragments lodging in the lungs and perforating the heart, permanent paralysis from the cement pressing on the spinal cord, and even deaths. Yet it's still unclear when, if ever, doctors will be convinced enough to stop using this treatment.

Understanding the science also shows how vertebroplasty could have initially appeared to be so miraculous. When the outcome being assessed is based upon patient judgment (pain, function, quality of sleep), studies that don't blind participants and investigators overestimate the treatment benefit by about an average of 25 per cent. This means that the results of the earlier studies of vertebroplasty are entirely consistent with the results from the placebo-controlled trials, as their estimate of benefit was about 25 per cent greater on average than the placebo-controlled trials.

Vertebroplasty is lucrative for the doctors who do it, as well as the device companies that provide the vertebroplasty kits (estimated to be worth $72 million in the North American market alone in 2016). It appears that they might go to any lengths to continue the practice. In a 2015 article in *The Atlantic* entitled 'The covert world of people trying to edit Wikipedia – for pay', journalist Joe Pinsker reports on the observations of Dr James Heilman, a Canadian emergency physician and a medical editor for Wikipedia. Heilman had found that the manufacturer, and one doctor who was heavily supported by the manufacturer, were attempting to alter the public record for vertebroplasty and the similar kyphoplasty (see chapter 8) in Wikipedia. The changes were being made to make the procedure look more favourable. One change was to add, after a statement that indicated that the procedures are 'controversial', the words 'among some but not among the actual physicians who perform these procedures'.

How can clinical observations be so wrong?

We've already seen the many reasons why it's difficult to change doctors' behaviour even in the face of overwhelming evidence.

The lack of respect for science comes from hubris or arrogance in doctors who think they know the answers when in fact their conclusions are flawed. It gets back to knowing and understanding science in the first place. But how can our observations have led us so astray? How is it possible to observe miraculous benefits of a treatment that later prove to be absent or not due to the treatment?

Our observations in the clinic are really no different from *observational* studies. We tend to treat everyone the same – there are no 'controls' – so it's not possible to truly know whether any observed improvement in an individual patient is actually a result of our treatment or would have occurred anyway, or with a different treatment.

Sometimes observational evidence is all you need, of course. You don't need to do a controlled experiment to see if parachutes are effective when jumping out of an aeroplane. This analogy is often used by critics of randomised trials to justify seemingly obvious treatment benefits but, unlike parachutes, it's rare for a medical condition to result in death immediately after diagnosis, and for the treatment to reverse that process immediately and save nearly every patient.

A review of publications where the parachute analogy was used to justify clinical practice found that randomised trials had actually been done to determine the value of about two-thirds of those practices. Only 27 per cent of these showed the practice to be beneficial. In 23 per cent of cases it was shown to be ineffective, and in another 23 per cent the results were mixed. For the rest, the trials were either halted or ongoing.

People find observational evidence very compelling. It's common for doctors to claim that more objective, experimental studies aren't required because they 'know' the treatment works. When the experimental evidence is produced, however, the results tend to be very sobering. In the famous study of citrus fruit for scurvy mentioned earlier, citrus was compared to many other treatments thought to be effective for scurvy (including sulfuric acid, sea water and vinegar). It took a study that used directly compared groups to convince people what worked and what didn't.

Doctors and patients can also be fooled into believing that the treatment has worked because many health problems, such as tennis elbow, headaches and influenza, are self-limiting, which means they improve over time without any treatment. This is known as the 'natural history' of the condition: what happens if we do nothing. This is why every treatment for the common cold and even an acute episode of non-serious low back pain *appears* to work – the appearance (observation) is an illusion that can be exposed and explained by science (experimental studies). People with both conditions improve over time and the treatment is irrelevant.

People usually seek medical help when their complaint is at its worst. For example, if you have recurring, fluctuating knee pain, you might go to the doctor when it has become intolerable. Chances are, the next time you see your doctor you will be better because your complaint is never *always* at its worst. This is called 'regression to the mean' or the tendency for extreme measures to go back to the average over time.

Another issue is placebo effects, sometimes called 'contextual' effects. In some trials, up to 60 per cent of the benefit that was observed could be explained by contextual effects, from such things as having an expectation that the treatment is going to work and having a caring believer in the treatment prescribing it. Contextual effects are also greater when you have more investment in the treatment working. If you paid a lot of money to get the treatment, for instance, you will be more ready to believe it works. Studies have shown that more invasive treatments, like injections or surgery, have a much greater placebo effect than taking a pill.

And more startling, even if you know you're receiving a placebo pill, you're still likely to benefit from its placebo effects. In a Portuguese randomised controlled trial of people with low back pain, half the participants were given a placebo pill. They were *told* it was a placebo pill and also *told* that this meant that the pill had no healing properties at all. Yet the group who knowingly took the placebo pill did better than those who weren't given the pill. In fact, after the study ended, some wanted to know where they could buy the placebo pills.

Numerous treatments that were initially heralded as breakthroughs later turned out to be ineffective, and we cover many in this book. It's important to point out that there's no inherent *harm* in that – medicine *should* be continuing to identify and test promising new treatments. Some will turn out to be genuine advances and many will not.

The problem arises when the 'breakthrough' treatment becomes part of usual care before it has been properly tested. It's much harder to disinvest from a treatment that has already become the standard

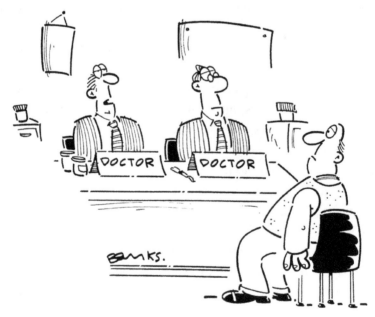

"ONE OF US IS A PLACEBO, MR JONES..."

of care, as in the case of vertebroplasty. In fact, while in some jurisdictions funding for this procedure has been withdrawn, in others it was determined to be too difficult to even try to withdraw funding for fear of a backlash from both doctors and the public.

Knee arthroscopy: a treatment whose time has passed

Knee arthroscopy, a procedure that involves inserting a camera and surgical instruments into the knee through small keyholes, is one of the most common surgical procedures in the world. It's commonly done for 'degeneration in the knee' – things like osteoarthritis, and cracks, splits and tears in the small cartilages called menisci.

Many studies published since the early 2000s have shown knee arthroscopy to be no more effective than placebo or exercise therapy for most conditions, yet the rates of surgery continued to rise throughout the 2000s. In the studies, patients in both groups largely improved, but those treated with arthroscopy didn't improve any *more* than those treated with the comparison treatment, or placebo surgery.

When surgeons see these improvements after performing knee arthroscopy for their patients with degenerative knees, it seems logical to them that the improvement was a direct result of their treatment. Because of the logical 'shortcut' humans make, observational evidence is very compelling for surgeons. It's very difficult for a surgeon (or any doctor) to accept experimental evidence that wasn't done on their patients, by them, particularly when they're unaware of the biases inherent in their own observations and of the power of the experimental evidence.

While the numbers of knee arthroscopies performed in some regions (such as Norway and Australia) have fallen significantly, in many countries and regions they have not, and in others they continue to rise. Yet even the falls that we have seen have only occurred since 2011, many years after the initial evidence was produced. It will probably take a few more decades for the rates to be anywhere near what they should be – for degenerative conditions, close to zero. Unfortunately, although change arises from weight of evidence, in the end change is still a social phenomenon, often relying on generations of doctors to change.

Surgery for shoulder tendons – redundant as well?

A similar scenario is now playing out in shoulder surgery. One of the most common surgical procedures for shoulder pain is a 'decompression' for presumed 'impingement' of the deep shoulder tendons (called the rotator cuff) as they pass between the shoulder joint and the bones above it. It involves an arthroscopy of the shoulder and shaving of some bone (acromioplasty) to stop it 'impinging' on the rotator cuff tendons. Two studies have now shown that surgery is no better than placebo surgery. The people in the placebo group received everything the surgery group did (i.e. the anaesthetic, surgical incisions, insertion of cameras and often other procedures) but not the acromioplasty.

Both placebo studies, one from the United Kingdom and one from Finland, made big news when published in 2018. But the procedure was already a topic of debate among shoulder specialists, many believing it offered no benefit and others believing it was valuable and often needed. Importantly, previous studies of the surgery compared with non-operative (exercise) controls had also shown that it was no more effective than non-surgical treatment. But it was only when the placebo studies were published that many surgeons sat up and took notice. Some were critical of the placebo studies, but the consistent findings across all the studies provide very compelling evidence that surgery offers no benefit.

It's often said that surgeons are often wrong but never in doubt. Many other operations are performed solely to relieve pain (rather than, say, cure cancer or appendicitis). Only a few have been compared to a placebo procedure, despite the clear advantages and ethical obligation to do such research where doubt exists. Unfortunately, that doubt rarely exists in the minds of the surgeons, whose attitude is reflected in these words from the philosopher Bertrand Russell: 'What [people] want is not knowledge but certainty'.

Shooting the messenger

It's one thing to lack respect for the science, but sometimes we disrespect the scientists. The history of medicine includes many examples of personal attacks and attempts to discredit scientists whose findings were unpopular or contrary to accepted beliefs. Semmelweis's demonstration of the value of antiseptic handwashing was widely rejected by the medical establishment in his lifetime. At the age of 47 he was committed to a lunatic asylum by his colleagues, allegedly suffering a nervous breakdown related to his insistence on believing and promoting his findings. He died two weeks later after being beaten by the guards.

From whatever angle, personal attacks on researchers whose findings are 'inconvenient', particularly when orchestrated by other doctors, seems an ultimate betrayal of the Hippocratic Oath.

Dr Michael E Mann, a distinguished scientist attacked for his work demonstrating that climate change is man-made, has dubbed this targeting of the messenger rather than taking on the science the 'Serengeti approach' – after the lions in the Serengeti who prey on the vulnerable zebras at the edge of the herd. In his own words, 'special interests faced with adverse scientific evidence ... target individual scientists rather than take on an entire scientific field at once'. Avoiding a genuine scientific discussion of the research by abusing the character or motive of the scientist making the argument is also a logical fallacy, termed an *ad hominem* ('to the person') attack.

Dr Barry Marshall: stomach ulcers

In the early to mid-1980s, Professor Barry Marshall, an Australian gastroenterologist, was widely ridiculed for his conviction that stomach ulcers were caused by bacteria and not by stress, too much spicy food or too much acid. Together with Professor Robin Warren, a pathologist, they discovered that the bacterium *Helicobacter pylori* plays a causal role in stomach ulcers. When they initially submitted their findings to the Gastroenterological Society of Australia, their paper was rejected. The reviewers had rated it in the bottom 10 per cent of papers they received in 1983. To prove the link, Professor Marshall even ingested a broth containing the bacterium and developed massive stomach inflammation three days later. After two decades, in 2005, once the Marshall and Warren theories were accepted and translated into the successful treatment of stomach ulcers, they received a Nobel Prize for their discovery.

The stakes are much higher when scientific evidence jeopardises powerful interest groups, as those campaigning against the harmful effects of smoking have found. Emeritus Professor Mike Daube, described in the *British Medical Journal* as 'probably Britain's pre-eminent health campaigner', has catalogued a long history of attempts to discredit people seen as threats by tobacco companies and their allies. Writing in the *Medical Journal of Australia* in 2015, he noted that 'Personal abuse and four-letter invective in blogs, tweets and emails are commonplace. Among the gentler comments, tobacco control leaders are liars, frauds, imbeciles, stupid, hate-filled, unethical, dishonest, hysterical, contemptible, insanely wicked, evil, sick, lunatics and paid tools of the pharmaceutical industry'.

Dr Bennet Omalu: chronic traumatic encephalopathy

Dr Bennet Omalu, a forensic pathologist, was one of the first people to recognise chronic traumatic encephalopathy in American football players. This condition, a form of dementia, is induced by repeated blows to the head, and had previously been identified in boxers. The NFL did not publicly acknowledge the link for seven years, during which time it mobilised experts on its payroll to discount Dr Omalu's work, and attempted to cover up the information.

A similar situation is now playing out in Australia. An article in the *New York Times* in 2019 indicated that more than 100 former Australian Rules football players have come forward and accused the AFL of attempting to avoid culpability for exposing the players to the known dangers of repeated concussions, as well as resisting calls to pay their medical costs. At the same time, the league has instigated concussion protocols for current players.

Chronic traumatic encephalopathy has now been confirmed in the brains of high-profile AFL players, as well as the brains of at least two former Australian rugby league players. A historic insurance payout of AU$1.4 million was recently made to former AFL footballer Shaun Smith, who played in the late 1980s and 1990s. He was found to be 'totally and permanently disabled' as a result of brain injuries he acquired playing the game.

Dr Sherine Gabriel: silicone breast implants

On the other side of the coin, scientists can also be harassed and intimidated when their results *fail* to confirm that a medical intervention is harmful. This happened to Professor Sherine Gabriel, a world-renowned rheumatologist. Professor Gabriel's offence was finding no link between silicone breast implants and the development of a range of autoimmune diseases in the first high-quality study to properly investigate this issue. Published in the *New England Journal of Medicine* in 1994, the study examined the medical records of all residents of Olmsted County in Minnesota from 1964 to 1991 and concluded that of the 749 women in the county with breast implants, not a single one had excess medical problems. Her findings were subsequently confirmed by many other studies.

These results were problematic because by then many multimillion-dollar awards had been made to women with breast implants on the basis that they were harmful, and many more were in the works. Professor Gabriel received death threats and other personal attacks for her work. Most of the personal attacks came from plaintiffs' lawyers, a powerful vested-interest group who were making money from the legal cases trying to show that the implants were causing health problems. The study had been conceived and designed by Professor Gabriel and her colleagues at the Mayo Clinic totally independent of vested interests, but several months after the study had started it did receive partial funding from the Plastic Surgery Educational Foundation, the educational arm of the American Society of Plastic Surgeons. While she knew the study findings might infuriate some people, she never dreamed she would be the victim of such vitriol.

The then editor-in-chief of the *New England Medical Journal*, Dr Marcia Angell, who was also harassed for allowing publication of the paper, noted in an accompanying editorial that the breast implant cases had been settled on the basis of case histories that by no means showed cause and effect, but had been accepted as nearly irrefutable truth. Dr Angell went on to write a book about the whole saga called *Science on Trial: The Clash of Medical Evidence and the Law in the Breast Implant Case*, published in 1996.

Personal attacks on us

We have both come under personal attack and been exposed to intimidation by other doctors for our advocacy of evidence-based medicine. Rachelle's troubles first started almost 20 years ago. In 2002, the week she published a paper in the prestigious *Journal of the American Medical Association* (*JAMA*), she opened her email to find a message from a complete stranger suggesting that she put her head in a microwave oven … and turn it on. Apparently, she had single-handedly ruined the lives of people with heel pain who would now be denied a miraculous cure. The crime? A trial finding that the treatment, shock-wave therapy, successfully used to break up kidney stones, was no better than placebo for heel pain. Unbeknown to her at the time, the publication coincided with FDA approval for this treatment in the United States, so the trial results put that decision into jeopardy. Several more emails followed, and one generously included a link to a blog devoted to countless conspiracy theories about Rachelle's motives.

The next episode involved the vertebroplasty trial and began well before the results were even known. True believers convinced by their personal experiences considered the trial unethical, and regularly shouted at and heckled Rachelle at professional meetings. From the day the trial results were published, she started to receive daily emails and calls from one vocal proponent of the treatment; letters of complaint about her were sent to the National Health and Medical Research Council, which had funded the trial, and to university leaders. The emails and phone calls ceased only after the university threatened legal action. Attempts to discredit Rachelle continued in other ways. For example, supporters of the procedure tried to stop the publication of her invited editorial in the *Medical Journal of Australia* and, when that failed, demanded that it be retracted.

Two years later, a further publication from Rachelle about vertebroplasty, published in the *British Medical Journal*, prompted a doctor from a prestigious US medical institution to copy her in on an email he had written to a device company. He complained that the paper had ruined things for him and he wouldn't be participating in any more vertebroplasty studies. He went on to suggest that she was a 'socialist charlatan, better suited to practise medicine in China or Cuba' but doubted that 'she would be given a licence in either of those countries'. He then said he hoped that she (as well as the principal investigator of the other placebo-controlled trial) would have a vertebral fracture and be denied the vertebroplasty procedure. In this particular instance, the email writer saw the errors of his ways after a strongly worded letter was sent to the CEO of his institution.

Another example from our own experience was a letter sent by a doctor to a group of colleagues, criticising us both for voicing our opinions about the evidence base for certain treatments for osteoarthritis. The writer's wrath was, however, mainly reserved for one of us – the one who isn't an orthopaedic surgeon. The letter complained about an editorial we had written in the *Medical Journal of Australia* and even our appearance on the ABC's flagship current affairs program *Four Corners* in a 2015 piece by Norman Swan and Joel Tozer titled 'Wasted', which exposed the waste in the health system and overdiagnosis. The letter went on to state that 'many … believe that having an academic rheumatologist give frequent and didactic advice about surgical management of knee osteoarthritis is an example of the Dunning-Kruger Effect'. People with this affliction have limited knowledge or competence on a given topic, dramatically overestimate their abilities and also lack insight into their own incompetence. This is a perfect example of an *ad hominem* attack that deflects attention from the actual issues.

These days, it's common for doctors to use social media sites such as Twitter and Facebook to promote new medical research findings and treatments (which, we guess, fulfils this chapter's pledge of the Hippocratic Oath to 'share hard-won scientific gains'). These platforms also make it easier to intimidate and misinform, which discourages many doctors from speaking out for science-based medicine. It's commonly the loudest and most shocking posts, not the most scientific, that spread the most.

Dr Alexandra Barratt: breast and prostate cancer screening

Professor Alex Barratt is a Sydney-based, internationally celebrated epidemiologist who has been studying, speaking and writing on cancer screening in a scientific, balanced and professional manner for 20 years. Her research has shown the downside of breast and prostate cancer screening, such as the high rate of overdiagnosed cancers ('harmless' cancers that would never have been found without screening) and false positive tests. Her work has found, for example, that about 20–30 per cent of breast cancers detected by screening are low-risk, non-progressive cancers.

Because she has exposed the failure of screening programs to acknowledge and communicate these problems, she has been called wrong, stupid, ill informed, dangerous and evil. She has been told that her words amount to killing people who may be dissuaded from breast and prostate cancer screening. A senior government medical adviser said she was irresponsible and should stop speaking publicly. An editor of one of the nation's leading medical journals asked her if she realised she would never get another cancer grant in her life. Others in senior positions in cancer agencies have declined her requests to work collaboratively on research to inform women of the risk of breast cancer overdiagnosis, refused to meet with her, blacklisted her from committees and marginalised her professionally.

Yet what she is advocating for – information for women and men about the main downside of screening, overdiagnosis – is now routinely included in information sent to UK women who are invited to breast cancer screening. This happened after an independent UK review of breast cancer screening in 2012 found that about 20 per cent of the breast cancers it picks up are overdiagnosed. Australian women are still waiting for information about overdiagnosis and overtreatment in their invitations for screening.

Professor Barratt's experience isn't unique. Both breast and prostate cancer screening (see chapter 3) are politicised and emotive topics. Raising scientific challenges to them has a long history of triggering controversy, which has often spilt over into the public domain. Other health professionals and journalists who have tried to tell the public about overdiagnosis in other countries have met similar resistance and have experienced enduring professional pressure and marginalisation.

Dr Minna Johansson: abdominal aortic aneurysms

The PhD topic of Dr Minna Johansson, a general practitioner in Sweden, related to abdominal aortic aneurysm, a localised enlargement of the aorta that most commonly affects men. While most aneurysms are small and will likely never cause symptoms or rupture, some do grow, and when they rupture the death rate is more than 80 per cent. If detected before they rupture, they can be repaired, but this also carries a 2–5 per cent risk of death. Since the 2000s, Sweden, the United Kingdom and the United States have had screening programs for this condition for men over 65. Smoking is a major risk factor for abdominal aortic aneurysms and for their growth. But as smoking rates have fallen, so have both the number of aneurysms and the number of aneurysms that rupture. This means that the risk–benefit ratio of screening is likely to have shifted.

Dr Johansson's PhD determined the rate of overdiagnosis from screening for abdominal aortic aneurysm. Her results questioned the ongoing value of screening, particularly in view of the decline in smoking rates. At the very least she has argued that there be full disclosure of both the potential benefits and potential harms from screening to the men being screened. These harms can include the side effects from unnecessary treatment, but also anxiety – worrying you might have a ticking timebomb inside you that could explode. From her first publication in 2014, she was accosted at scientific meetings with comments like 'Think about all the men you have killed. How can you sleep at night?' She also describes receiving terrifying anonymous hate mail with extreme sexist content.

Professors of vascular surgery also used their academic power to try to prevent her from being awarded a PhD. They accused her of research fraud and made personal attacks, such as she is a 'fanatic with a religious conviction against screening'. They spread these accusations in a letter to influential people within academia in Sweden. Even after she was awarded her PhD and moved on to a new research position, they contacted her future boss to question her employment. There have been no consequences for the doctors concerned.

When science gets it wrong

To paraphrase Winston Churchill, science is the worst way of knowing, except for all the others. It's messy and it's hard, but it's still the best we've got.

A 2012 article in the journal *Nature* reported an attempt by researchers to independently replicate 53 landmark or breakthrough papers in the field of preclinical cancer research. Basically, they took these famous experimental studies and tried to repeat the original experiments, using the same ingredients and techniques, to see if they got the same results. The idea is that if scientific experiments are true, they should be reproducible, otherwise they're not much use to anyone and shouldn't be relied upon.

The authors found that, despite performing the original 53 experiments faithfully, often multiple times each, they could only reproduce the findings of six of them. They even went to the extent of contacting the original authors to make sure they were doing it right.

In one case, the original researcher wasn't surprised that his findings weren't reproducible, because it took him dozens of attempts to get the result he eventually published. In other words, he kept doing the experiment until one day he fluked the results he wanted and then published them, with no reference to all the times it failed. This kind of selective reporting of results is only part of the reproducibility problem in research. But whether it's selective reporting of results, selective inclusion of some data and exclusion of other data, or choosing the statistical methods that give the desired result, the problem stems from bias among the researchers. They may want to report newsworthy findings, get closer to a cure, win a prize, justify their funding or get more funding or a promotion. Whatever the reason, as soon as one type of result becomes more desirable to them than another, they will (consciously or subconsciously) try to achieve that result, instead of being objective and scientific, and letting the chips fall where they may.

The public's view of researchers is probably one of strictly scientific, objective people who would never tamper with their studies. We have both been performing research for a long time, often publishing in those top journals, and we agree that most researchers are well intentioned and unlikely to deliberately tamper with or falsify the results of a study. But we also know the results of a study can be presented, interpreted and adjusted in many ways. It can be very tempting, when faced with these myriad decisions about a study, to make the decision that's more likely to lead to the result you want. This is bias in research, and it leaks into studies wherever it can.

A 2005 review looking at the biggest studies published in the top general medical journals in the world found that most of them were either never replicated, or, when they were, yielded different results.

Some of the research listed in the 2012 *Nature* article that could not be reproduced had spawned new branches of research founded on the original (wrong) findings. Renowned sceptic and family physician and US Air Force surgeon Dr Harriet Hall has termed this 'tooth-fairy science' – a branch of science that studies a phenomenon without first establishing whether the phenomenon exists. It comes from mistaking evidence that is *consistent with* a theory for evidence that *confirms* a theory. A lot of research could be done about the tooth-fairy phenomenon itself: does the amount of money received vary for different teeth, or with different ways of leaving the tooth out for the fairy? Considerable data could be generated and correlations formed, and conferences could be convened to discuss the studies, but none of it would confirm the existence of a tooth fairy – that's just the assumption upon which all the research is based. This humorous example is only one step away from those who study UFOs, or alternatives to medicine, or many aspects of medicine.

These issues are well known and accepted among scientists but poorly understood by non-scientists: science often gets it wrong. We know this because it has been shown scientifically, and this is the point: the scientific method *isn't* wrong, but it often gives us wrong answers because we didn't *use* it right.

Science is like a set of tools to construct something. The 'something' we construct is an estimate of the truth, and the tools we use are those that minimise error. By minimising the error in our studies, we literally get the 'least wrong' answer. For trials, these tools include making sure we have enough participants to be sure of our results (sample size), randomisation (which helps us achieve two comparison groups that are similar at the start of the study) and blinding (which helps us ensure that, apart from the study treatment, both groups are treated equally). There are many other tools as well. But in the end, some trials are too small, some don't randomise well (or at all), and in some the treatment group of the participants is known (unblinding). This doesn't mean the tools are bad, it just means they weren't used properly – or not at all.

Using the science toolbox doesn't always give the right answer, but if you use the tools correctly it does give you the answer that's least likely to be wrong – it gives you the most *reliable* answer or the *best* estimate of the truth.

Yet people who find fault with clinical research often conclude that clinical research (science) itself is bad. But if somebody builds a house badly, you don't blame the carpenter's tools or say that carpentry isn't a good way of constructing things. You just say they didn't *do it* well.

Some people have been critical of randomisation as a tool, claiming, for example, that it doesn't always result in the two comparison groups being perfectly matched, which might influence the results. This is true (for example, when you toss a coin ten times, you don't always get exactly five heads and five tails), but you should see how badly matched the patient groups are when they're *not* randomised! Randomisation is simply the fairest (least biased) way of dividing up participants in a trial. It often results in some differences between groups. This is called 'random error'. Scientists know about it and have standardised methods to minimise it.

When doctors criticise scientific studies (preferring instead to trust their own observations), we must ask what alternative they are offering. These critics say that science is often wrong so we can't *trust* it and shouldn't rely on it, but they offer no alternative, except perhaps for us to trust *them*, their opinion.

The harshest critics of clinical trials, however, are the scientists who do the research that exposes true flaws in the methods. They all give the same solution: do the science better. They say that trials should include more people and include people who are more representative of the general population. They insist on proper randomisation and on blinding everyone: the patient, the doctor, the person administering the surveys and the statisticians doing the analysis. The *informed* critics of clinical research aren't saying that clinical research or science as a tool is bad, just that it needs to be *done* better.

* * *

Science (and the people doing it) should be respected. A careful and objective analysis gives us a better estimate of how well treatments work compared with relying on our experience or the experience of others. Science isn't always done well, but understanding it can help us better choose the evidence on which to base our decisions.

3

Overtreatment

Hippocratic Oath: I will apply, for the benefit of the sick, all measures which are required, avoiding those twin traps of overtreatment and therapeutic nihilism.

'Natural forces within us are the true healers of disease'
– attributed to Hippocrates

'I firmly believe that if the whole material medica, as now used, could be sunk to the bottom of the sea, it would be better for mankind, and all the worse for the fishes'
– Oliver Wendell Holmes, American physician and poet

One of the most telling illustrations of overtreatment took place in New York in the 1930s. Removing children's tonsils used to be a common procedure, performed for a variety of reasons, such as recurrent tonsillitis and breathing problems, but the practice varied widely between geographic regions and surgeons.

Researchers took a random sample of 1000 children. Noting that 60 per cent had already had their tonsils out, they sent the remaining 40 per cent to doctors to see if they should have their tonsils out too. Tonsillectomy was recommended in 45 per cent of those children. Just to make sure nobody was being undertreated, they did the same thing again, sending the remaining children to another group of doctors for a second opinion. Those doctors recommended tonsillectomy in 40 per cent of those children.

Yet again, the few children now remaining were sent to another group of doctors. This time, 44 per cent were recommended tonsillectomy. In the end, nearly all of the 1000 children either had a tonsillectomy or had one recommended. What were these doctors basing their decisions on? Possibly, they were thinking that about half of all kids need their tonsils out (not true, of course, but that was the thinking at the time) and they were just applying that belief as best they could, trying to pick the half that would be most likely to benefit.

Where's the harm in that? Tonsillectomy never killed anyone, right? Wrong: more than one in 30 patients are readmitted to hospital after tonsillectomy because of complications of the surgery, and about one in 15 000 will die as a result of the surgery. These rates were probably a lot worse back then, so we had a situation where the procedure was not only unnecessary in most cases but also potentially harmful.

From therapeutic nihilism to overtreatment

When treating any condition, there's a 'sweet spot' between believing everything works, and therefore overtreating people, and therapeutic nihilism – the idea that nothing works. Medicine today is at the 'overtreatment' end of this spectrum, but this wasn't always the case. Until the 19th century, many people thought that medicine did more harm than good. They believed instead that the most potent treatment was to allow the body to heal itself. One notable sceptic, Voltaire, famously said 'The art of medicine consists of amusing the patient while nature cures the disease'. Yet doctors were held in high regard by many because of their firm belief in the largely ineffective treatments of the time.

The notion of therapeutic nihilism faded in the 20th century after the introduction of an increasing number of effective treatments, such as vitamin C for scurvy, vitamin D to prevent or cure rickets, antibiotics for acute infections, and insulin for diabetes. But the concept resurfaced in the late 20th century in the writings of such people as the philosopher and social critic Ivan Illich. His 1975 book, *Limits to Medicine*, claimed that improvements in health and life expectancy were largely due to sanitation, nutrition and public health programs, and that individual treatments given by doctors resulted in net harm: 'the medical establishment has become a major threat to health'.

Much of his argument is that pain, suffering and death are part of life, and by taking over control of these aspects of life, medicine has diminished the capacity of people to cope. Illich coined the term 'iatrogenic' harm, referring to the physical and mental harms that can arise from medical care itself, particularly in the context of medicalising normal life.

There's merit in the notion that the huge improvements in life expectancy we have witnessed over the last few hundred years were due not so much to improvements in medical care applied to individuals but to social and political changes. The latter have allowed large-scale public policy and industrial revolutions, leading to availability of clean drinking water, wastewater separation and treatment, greater food availability through agricultural improvements, better food preparation and storage including refrigeration, fewer wars and declining rates of poverty.

Overtreatment: too much health care

Although there are now many useful tests and effective medical treatments, that doesn't mean *all* medical tests and treatments are effective, or that *every* complaint should be diagnosed and treated. Overtreatment is rampant in medicine and is arguably one of the largest problems in health care today. A 2011 study estimated that unnecessary services added US$158–226 billion per year to US healthcare spending. More recently, in Washington state alone, a report from 2018 (aptly titled *First, Do No Harm*) estimated that 600 000 people each year had treatment they didn't need, costing more than US$280 million.

Each year in Australia, billions of dollars are spent on medical tests, procedures and treatments that don't make us any healthier and sometimes make us worse off. The *Australian Financial Review* estimates that federal and state governments and private health insurers alone pay about AU$30 billion for ineffective or unwarranted care every year.

This problem of overtreatment has also been highlighted in series by several leading medical journals, including the *British Medical Journal*'s popular 'Too Much Medicine', *JAMA*'s 'Less is More' and the *Journal of Hospital Medicine*'s 'Things We Do for No Reason'. In Australia, a collaboration of academics from around the country have called for a national action plan to address overdiagnosis and overtreatment.

Overtreatment, in the broadest sense, means 'too much health care'. This covers a whole spectrum of inappropriate care, from too much testing, to too much diagnosis and too much treatment. It occurs both in people with symptoms and healthy people without symptoms. The hallmark of too much health care is that not only does it provide no worthwhile benefit, but it might cause harm – in other words, it does more harm than good.

Overtreatment takes many forms. Many invasive and uncomfortable yet futile treatments are applied to people who are dying, denying them of a dignified and comfortable death. Healthy people who have nothing wrong with them can also be given unnecessary treatments that provide no health improvements but still carry risks.

The problem of unnecessary care is no secret to doctors. In a survey of US doctors, physicians felt that around 20 per cent of all medical care was unnecessary, including 25 per cent of all tests and 11 per cent of all procedures. Most of the respondents felt that the problem was partly due to doctors profiting from the procedures. This was coming from the doctors themselves, but given that doctors overestimate the benefits of their treatments and underestimate the harms, the real estimate of unnecessary care is likely to be much higher.

More objective reports confirm this. Of the US$750 billion estimated to be wasted in the US health system in 2010, the largest category of excess costs was unnecessary services at $210 billion. The total amount of excess costs makes up more than 30 per cent of the total costs of health care in the United States, and health care makes up around 18 per cent of the gross domestic product (GDP). This means that waste in the healthcare system accounts for more than 5 per cent of the US GDP.

The news from other countries isn't much better. The OECD, which includes 37 member countries across the globe, estimates that about one-fifth of healthcare spending is wasted. This is equivalent to more than US$1 trillion annually. The WHO also estimates healthcare waste at 20–40 per cent of total expenditure. A 2019 study investigating the extent of overuse in medical care in Australian hospitals found that in two-thirds of relevant studies, the estimate of overuse exceeded 30 per cent.

Fixing heart plumbing: cardiac stenting

One of the most common procedures in medicine is cardiac stenting, which is worth billions to the medical and device industries. The procedure involves inserting a stiff metal tube into a narrowed heart artery to widen it. The stent is normally inserted under X-ray control, fed in from a blood vessel in the groin or arm. On the face of it, it makes sense to try to widen or unblock a narrowed artery just as you would a water or sewerage pipe that was blocked, and doctors have become very good at it. They can even pass a stent up through a completely blocked artery. The procedure is often done on patients in whom a narrowed blood vessel has been found using angiography (injecting dye into the bloodstream and X-raying the arteries). The patient may have had symptoms but not necessarily a heart attack and sometimes they haven't had symptoms at all. The temptation to open a narrowed artery is very strong; it just seems to make so much sense.

Sometimes, however, things that seem straightforward and logical at first start to lose their appeal on closer inspection. For example, if the patient wasn't having a heart attack and they already had a completely (or near completely) blocked vessel, how was their heart still working? Does the blood find its way in through other channels that have opened up because of the blockage? What happens to the stents – do they block up again? What are the possible complications from having the procedure? What about the anticoagulant drugs that need to be taken for life to stop the stent from blocking – do they cause complications, like bleeding?

To try to prevent the stents blocking up again, people need to take lifelong blood-thinning medication, which can cause bleeding. If left to its own devices, the body can also adapt to the narrowing by opening up other arteries, called collateral circulation. There's even evidence that the narrowest vessels seen on an angiogram aren't the ones that block up in a heart attack, and that the severity of narrowing is not associated with how soon a heart attack may occur. If the narrowed vessel isn't the problem, this seems to be another example of 'tooth-fairy science'.

The simplest and most important question, though, for this and any other procedure in medicine, is this: is doing the procedure better for the patient than not doing it? What would have happened had the stent not been inserted? One way to answer that question is to do a controlled study with two groups – to insert stents in some people and not insert them in others. This exact study, called the COURAGE trial, was published in 2007, and involved people who would commonly be treated with a stent. It randomly divided more than 2000 patients with severe coronary artery disease who had 'stable angina' (episodic chest pain but not an acute heart attack) into a stent group and a no-stent group. Both groups received best medical care comprising the usual drug treatment. The results showed that stenting offered no additional benefit over good medical treatment (the drugs) alone. The participants knew exactly which treatment they had received, as did the people who were following them up. Yet even with this knowledge, people who had received the stents did not fare any better. They did not die less often or have fewer heart attacks. Despite these results, clinical practice didn't change much. Doctors argued that although stenting might not reduce the chances of dying or having a heart attack, it still might reduce episodes of angina (episodic chest pain).

After *years* of continued stenting of *millions* of people with known coronary artery disease but stable angina, an even better type of study was published in 2017, a randomised placebo-controlled trial called ORBITA. It included the same type of patients as the COURAGE trial – those with severe narrowing of the coronary arteries and stable angina. But this time the doctors gave one group of patients a stent, and *pretended* to give the other group a stent (i.e. a placebo). The groups were assigned at random and neither the patients nor the people providing the follow-up care knew who got what. This means they avoided the influence of expectations for a given treatment. This time the outcome they were most interested in was symptoms such as how long the patients could exercise for and how frequent were their episodes of chest pain. As in the other trial, stenting did not help any more than the pretend stenting for any of the outcomes measured.

A further trial comparing stenting to medical care without stenting in more than 5000 people with moderate or severe heart disease was published in 2020. It also showed no difference in the outcomes between the two groups. While not all stents are currently performed for people with stable angina, many are. It's estimated that tens of thousands of cardiac stent procedures performed each year in the United States are unnecessary, at a cost of billions of dollars.

The ongoing debate about the value of stenting in people with coronary artery disease and stable angina has led to some interesting developments. Hospitals and doctors in the United States have been penalised under the False Claims Act for defrauding the government by charging Medicare for this unnecessary care. This is very rare in medicine, but it's worth noting that hospitals investigated under this Act decreased stenting at a greater rate than did similar hospitals that weren't charged with fraud. Despite all the evidence and the penalties, however, the rates of unhelpful and costly cardiac stenting remain high internationally.

We can't all be right

Sometimes overtreatment can be detected by practice variation, differences in the use of certain tests or treatments between different regions, or different hospitals or individual doctors, that isn't explained by differences between the populations being served. Studies of practice variation have shown high rates of unexplained variation in the use of surgery, including common operations such as gallbladder removal, spinal fusion and cardiac stents; antibiotic prescribing; and even unexpected things like kidney dialysis. Even within these treatments there is variation. For example, the use of dialysis in patients with kidney failure varies, as do the rates of blood transfusion in dialysis patients, the frequency of dialysis and even the threshold for starting dialysis; and these variations cannot be explained by medical need. Various editions of the *Australian Atlas of Health Care Variation* have identified many signals of overuse of tests and treatments in Australia. These include cardiac and thyroid tests; CT scans and surgery of the lumbar spine; early planned caesarean sections; gastroscopies and colonoscopies; knee replacements and knee arthroscopy; antibiotic dispensing to adults and children; prescription; and opioid, antidepressant and other prescriptions for mental health.

Many studies of practice variation are done within countries, but the variation *between* countries can be even worse. For example, the rate of spinal fusion surgery in the United States is nearly ten times higher than in the United Kingdom. The problem with studies of practice variation, however, is that they don't tell you who's right. Without knowing the *appropriate* rate of treatment, we don't know if, using the spinal fusion example, the rate in the United States is too high, if the rate in Britain is too low, or both. What practice variation does tell us though (given there's no other explanation for the variation) is that *someone* is wrong.

Unwarranted practice variation may occur for many reasons. Often it's simply due to uncertainty. Doctors aren't sure how effective a certain treatment is, and no high-quality evidence yet exists to guide them. It can also be due to different teachings and to local doctor preferences and beliefs. Financial incentives, or the lack of them, can explain the differences too. For example, in the United States, surgeons are paid very well for spinal fusion surgery but in the United Kingdom's public health system, surgeons make no more or less money whether they treat patients with or without surgery.

Unfortunately, financial incentives may also lead to the use of more costly alternative treatments that not only fail to offer benefits over lower-priced services, but may also cause harm. We know that the number of complex fusion surgeries (where many vertebrae in the spine are fused together) for spinal stenosis, a narrowing of the spinal canal that commonly occurs with age, is growing at a rapid rate in the United States, Australia, Norway and many other developed countries. We also know that it's three times more expensive than the simpler 'decompression' procedure, which widens the narrowed spinal canal without fusing the vertebrae together. Trials have shown that the addition of fusion to decompression alone not only has negligible if any health benefits, but also doubles the chance of wound complications and increases the rate of strokes and deaths within 30 days of the operation.

Is it possible to have too many tests?

Too many tests are a big part of unnecessary care: blood and other pathology tests, imaging studies and sometimes even checking someone's blood pressure when it isn't warranted. A commonly cited reason for overtesting is that doctors don't want to miss anything serious. Doctors are taught to be on the lookout for 'red flags', clues in the patient's history or physical examination that might indicate something sinister. This is appropriate and an expected part of the doctor's job. But doing tests when there's no compelling suspicion of serious disease or 'just to be sure' is leading doctors astray. This fear of missing something is related to the fear of malpractice lawsuits, which has led to so-called 'defensive medicine', typically characterised by performing excessive tests. A 2010 study estimated that US$55.6 billion, or 2.4 per cent of the total US healthcare spend, could be attributed to medical liability costs, including defensive medicine.

While some tests such as X-rays and CT scans expose patients to radiation and even taking blood can cause localised bruising, the tests themselves often result in very little direct physical harm. But harms may arise from what the tests discover. There's a very good chance that a test will detect something 'abnormal' when it's really either falsely abnormal – that is, a 'false-positive' result – or something altogether harmless that didn't *need* to be found. One Canadian study estimated that more than half the laboratory tests performed by family doctors (general practitioners) could give false-positive results. This seems incredibly high but can be explained.

Most laboratory tests have a range of values considered to lie within the 'normal range' rather than a specific cut-off between normal and abnormal, and this can vary with age, gender and population as well as in the way the test is performed. Let's consider the normal level of haemoglobin, the substance in blood that carries oxygen around the body. The normal range in Australia, according to the Australian Red Cross, is between 130 and 180 g/L in men and between 120 and 160 g/L in women. This normal range, which has been determined by looking at the spread of values in a group of healthy people, indicates the levels that most people (95 per cent) have. Five per cent of healthy, normal people will therefore have values that fall either above or below that range even though there's nothing wrong with them. To put it another way, if 100 healthy people are tested, five of them will have results that fall outside what's considered to be the 'normal' range.

The more tests you do on healthy people, the more of them will be falsely positive. Being more selective with who we test, by only doing tests when we have a high suspicion that something is wrong, reduces the risk of false-positive tests. This rule also applies to imaging tests. There are some 'normal' ranges in imaging, such as the size a mass in the lung must be before it's considered abnormal and requiring further investigation to exclude it being a cancer. But the biggest problem for imaging is finding lots of abnormalities, sometimes called 'incidentalomas', that are likely normal for a person's age, so they're not exactly false positives but changes that are of no concern at all.

In both situations, having a false-positive test and finding 'something' that's really harmless (in other words, nothing), can be costly and can cause unnecessary anxiety and psychological harm. It can also lead to significant downstream physical harms if the non-existent condition is treated.

Unnecessary imaging for low back pain

A common fallacy is that people with low back pain need imaging to identify the precise cause of the pain so that the right treatment can be prescribed. More than 60 per cent of patients and at least a third of doctors believe this, but imaging is likely to find lots of abnormalities (e.g. bulging discs, osteoarthritis and narrowed nerve canals). And finding them is likely to result in overtreatment.

Even with the advent of increasingly sensitive tests such as CT scans and MRI scans, in the majority of cases we cannot identify the precise cause of the problem. Various abnormalities detected in these imaging tests, especially the more advanced types of imaging, are extremely common in people without back pain. They also increase with age, so many simply reflect normal age-related changes. While some of these abnormalities may be associated with the presence of pain, there is no way of knowing whether they are the cause of the problem in an individual patient or just incidental.

Knowing that these abnormalities are present may not actually help either, as the treatment is usually the same regardless of the imaging findings. In fact, most people who have an episode of pain get better quickly, and this happens irrespective of any treatment. Overall, less than 1 per cent of people who visit their GP with acute low back pain will have a serious cause for their pain, and even in the emergency department that rate is less than 5 per cent.

The reality is that many people with low back pain get imaging when they don't really need it. Considering that most of us will have back pain at some time or another, and about half of us will be sufficiently worried to see a doctor, that's a lot of unnecessary imaging. To try to ascertain the exact proportion of unnecessary imaging and whether this had changed over time, we recently compiled all the studies that had reported imaging for patients with low back pain presenting to either their GP or to the emergency department in the two decades from 1995 to 2015. We found 45 studies from nine countries reporting on more than 19 million consultations for low back pain. One in four patients attending their GP were referred for imaging, and this rose to one in three in the emergency department (which makes sense, as people who go there generally have more pain). Furthermore, the chances of having a more sensitive and expensive test, such as a CT or MRI scan rather than a plain X-ray, increased by more than 50 per cent over that time period.

But where's the harm in having your back scanned? Surely it's better to know exactly what's going on and make sure it's nothing serious. For some people this might be reassuring, but for many

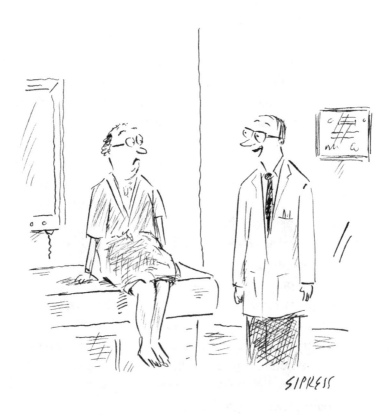

"I can cure your back problem, but there's a risk that you'll be left with nothing to talk about."

it's likely to be a source of more anxiety rather than less. When minimal abnormalities are found, people with severe symptoms might be left wondering how this can be possible and worry that the doctor and others will think they are exaggerating their pain or even making it up. In others, unwarranted imaging of the spine not only exposes them to unnecessary radiation if they have an X-ray or CT scan, it's also likely to lead to unnecessary treatments, including opioid prescriptions and surgery.

For example, while a CT or MRI scan might show a bulging disc in the spine, this diagnosis is unhelpful, as almost all people develop bulging discs as they age, and it might have nothing whatsoever to do with the pain. A doctor might think it does, though, and prescribe strong pain medication, or they might refer the patient to a surgeon, who may in turn offer the patient surgery. The more advanced the imaging, the more likely it will find abnormalities, so the greater the chances of being overtreated for no gain. A trial performed in the United States in people first visiting their doctor with low back pain randomised half of the group to have an MRI scan and the other half to have an X-ray. At the end of 12 months both groups had exactly the same outcomes, but the group who had the MRI scans were more than twice as likely to have had an operation.

Why do doctors do too many tests?

After fear of being sued, the second most common reason surveyed US doctors knowingly order unnecessary tests is that the patients request them. While it's highly likely that doctors overestimate how much care patients really want, there's no doubt that changes in societal norms have led to more demands for tests by patients. Some of this has been driven by overzealous selling of the value of tests by vested interests. But as in the low back pain example, some of this is driven by misconceptions among both clinicians and the general public about the value of different tests. Both often overestimate the benefits, but are less aware of the potential harms. Part of the blame rests with doctors, who may not routinely explain potential harms of testing to their patients, and may also see value in information for its own sake.

The public's perspective

Studies have found that the public are largely unaware of the concepts of overtesting and overdiagnosis or understand them poorly. While people understand the concept of overtreatment, they have faith in testing and cannot see the harm. They don't recognise that unnecessary testing can lead to overdiagnosis, which might in turn lead to overtreatment. They consider that the decision-making about their care starts *after* the test or series of tests, not *before*. Because they see inherent value in *any* information about their bodies, they are much more sceptical and less receptive of the need to reduce overtesting.

Incidental abnormalities can cause worry in both the doctor and the patient. A recent study found that even in the *absence* of symptoms, more than 50 per cent of patients would choose to undergo high-risk surgery based on abnormalities detected by imaging their spine.

Another problem is the overtesting that occurs as a matter of routine, often in the context of being admitted to hospital or having an operation. Batteries of tests are routinely ordered before surgery, but many of these are unnecessary. Similarly, a panel of blood tests and imaging may be done almost routinely on arrival in an emergency department, regardless of the reason the person attended.

While overtesting and overdiagnosis are not the same thing (you can have overdiagnosis without overtesting, as explained below), the more tests you have, the greater your risk of being overdiagnosed or receiving an unnecessary diagnosis. This is exactly what's likely to happen if you undergo a comprehensive full-body health check-up.

Full-body health checks: discovering 'hidden problems'

Full-body health checks are often offered to company executives, or directly advertised to the general public, for example through newspaper advertorials. They might even feature in the health report on television news programs. As well as a comprehensive clinical evaluation, the 'check-up' usually involves having a battery of laboratory tests, often including genetic tests (see below) and advanced imaging. It's offered for a set fee, which in Australia is upwards of AU$2000. The cost is borne entirely by the patient (or the company), as it's generally not covered by health insurance. And the fee doesn't cover the additional costs of the almost inevitable follow-up tests and treatments.

Most, if not all people who have these check-ups don't feel ill. They're usually convinced by the promise that these checks can identify serious medical conditions early, and that you will be taking control of your health and gaining peace of mind. Unfortunately, these are false promises. Not only are these checks unlikely to be beneficial, but they entail myriad potential harms. If they fail to detect serious illness, they may provide false reassurance. Imagine smokers being told they are healthy. They might then decide it's unnecessary to quit smoking. Having the test itself can be fatal, as illustrated by the 2019 death of a healthy Australian woman who had an anaphylactic reaction to contrast dye injected as part of a heart scan her employer suggested she have.

More alarming is the fact that it's likely to identify 'hidden problems'. HealthScreen, one company offering these types of full body checks in Australia, for example, has claimed that 'so far the doctors have found hidden problems in every patient'.

This is especially true the more extensive the check-up. These so-called hidden problems are usually overdiagnoses that can lead to detrimental psychological effects, unnecessary further tests and unnecessary treatment.

Bogus screening programs and direct advertising

Occasionally doctors who are a little less scrupulous about their oath set up screening services in areas not even debated in academic circles, because they are bogus. These are the shopping mall outfits offering whole-body CT scans, heel-pad density scans, gait measurements and various blood tests. The business model is simple but effective: the test can be done immediately with no pain and little or no cost to the individual. Like the full-body checks, they attract customers with a hook: without the test you don't know – with the test you do. But while these tests sound like a good idea, they don't satisfy the necessary criteria for effective screening. They can provide false reassurance, lead to harm (the radiation from whole-body CT scans affects many organs) and can alter the person's insurance risk.

Direct-to-consumer advertising, which is illegal in some countries, involves buying ad time on the media to inform the public about specific tests and treatments. The business model has one simple aim: to sell more product. A review of the evidence showed that it achieves its goal: it leads to an increase in the prescribing of the advertised drug or test. It also leads to more diagnoses, but not to health gains. The review didn't even consider the harms of the advertising, such as labelling people as diseased, or the harms from the treatments.

Personalised medicine

The public are now being sold the idea of having their genetic material mapped. The idea is that if doctors know your genetic make-up, they can detect abnormalities early and treat them, and this treatment can be 'personalised'.

'Personalised medicine' (or 'precision' medicine) was seen as a natural consequence of the mapping of the human genome in the late 1990s. In 2000, people were predicting that mapping the genetic make-up of individuals would enable prediction, diagnosis and treatment of many conditions, and would revolutionise the way medicine is practised within ten to 20 years. Yet although we can map a person's genome for no greater cost than many other medical tests, the touted benefits have not arrived. Apart from very few exceptions, diseases are not explained by a single gene variant; they are much more complicated and are mostly the result of a complex interaction between many genes and the environment. This means that identifying the risk of a certain disease or response to treatment with any degree of 'precision' has largely failed.

Yet the business of personalised medicine has thrived, supported by hype, our desire to see it work and the appeal of its simplistic model. It has become popular in the absence of a clear benefit to healthy people.

Overdiagnosis

The main reason we go to the doctor is for an explanation of the cause of our complaints, what the likely outcome might be, and advice on best management. The doctor gathers information from the patient's history and physical examination, and sometimes from things like blood tests or X-rays and scans. They then make a diagnosis, and advise appropriate treatment that benefits the patient. Sometimes, however, they give an unnecessary diagnosis that won't benefit the patient and might cause harm – this is 'overdiagnosis'.

The unnecessary diagnosis can be made with or without too many tests or 'overtesting'.

It's important to draw a distinction between *overdiagnosis* and *misdiagnosis*. *Mis*diagnosis is a *wrong* diagnosis – for example making a diagnosis of cancer when no cancer exists. But in *over*diagnosis, the diagnosis is *correct* – for example, the cancer really exists, but it's so small or slow growing that it would never have been noticed in the person's lifetime. In overdiagnosis, the diagnosis, and any consequent intervention, does not improve the outcome for the patient.

The distinction between *over*diagnosis and *mis*diagnosis becomes a bit trickier for non-cancer conditions. More sensitive tests, which sound better in theory, can actually result in *mis*diagnosis. For example, ultrasensitive tests for troponin (a heart muscle enzyme that leaks into the bloodstream when the heart is damaged) will show elevated troponin levels in many normal people, which might be misconstrued as meaning they've had a heart attack. More sensitive tests can also result in *over*diagnosis. High-resolution CT angiography might detect small emboli (clots) in very small arteries in the lungs. These clots are so small that radiologists disagree as to which ones could be a problem and which are within 'normal'. Many more clots are now being detected, but although these may never cause harm, the doctor feels compelled to treat the patient with blood-thinning medicines, which can cause their own complications, such as internal bleeding.

In a more recent example, a 2017 study performed in São Paulo, Brazil (and involving Rachelle) took more than 500 patients who had been recommended spinal surgery and invited them to seek a second opinion. The second opinion recommended surgery for only a third of the 92 per cent of patients who took up the offer, and in many of these cases the second doctor recommended a different operation. In fact, there was full agreement between the first and second opinions in only 15 per cent of cases. The remaining two-thirds of patients were advised not to have surgery at all, and about one in ten of these were thought not even to have a spinal condition. This discord between first and second opinions has been replicated in numerous other studies. The take-home message is that if a surgeon suggests spinal surgery – or a tonsillectomy – it would be prudent to seek a second opinion.

Screening for cancer in well people

Screening is a strategy used to identify the presence of an as-yet-undiagnosed disease in people with no signs or symptoms. The premise is that picking up the condition early will lead to better outcomes than if the condition is discovered later. This of course depends upon having effective treatments to treat or cure the condition in the first place. If there's no effective treatment, then screening for an incurable disease just means that you live longer with the knowledge of having it but not being able to do anything about it.

But what if the condition would *never* have caused symptoms or harm if it had been left undetected and untreated? This is one of the defining characteristics of overdiagnosis. People are given a diagnosis that labels them with a condition and the diagnosis is correct (it's not a 'false positive' or misdiagnosis), but neither the diagnosis nor any consequent intervention improve the outcome for the patient.

Much of the focus on overdiagnosis from testing has been for cancer, such as prostate specific antigen (PSA) testing for prostate cancer, ultrasound scans for thyroid cancer, and chest X-rays for lung cancer. The problem is that these tests may not detect the severe cancers that kill people, which because they grow rapidly and lead to death quickly are unlikely to be 'caught' at the moment of screening. But screening will detect milder forms of cancer, which are growing at a moderate pace, or more slowly, or sometimes not even growing at all. It might also detect abnormalities that are precursors for cancer.

Not all of them will *become* cancer but they might be diagnosed as 'early' or 'precancerous' conditions.

This means that many people are being unnecessarily diagnosed and treated, with accompanying harms and costs, for no net benefit. It has been estimated that 18000 cancers in men and 11000 in women may be overdiagnosed each year in Australia. This represents about 24 per cent of cancers diagnosed in men and 18 per cent of cancers diagnosed in women each year. Overdiagnosed cancers include mainly the ones that are non-invasive, possibly due to the increasing popularity of skin checks, kidney cancer (incidentally picked up on CT scans done for other reasons) and thyroid cancers. But the greatest numbers are in prostate cancer in men (more than 8500 a year) and breast cancers in women (almost 4000 a year). Similar rates have been observed in other countries. In the United States it has been estimated that 70000 women are overdiagnosed with breast cancer each year.

Mass screening for thyroid cancer

Overdiagnosis of thyroid cancer is possibly the best example of how mass screening for cancer can go wrong. Papillary thyroid cancer is a common but frequently inactive form of thyroid cancer. Due to mass screening it's being diagnosed in record numbers.

A 2017 study from Switzerland showed a doubling in the diagnosis of thyroid cancer for women (per population) between 1998 and 2012, and an associated four-fold increase in thyroidectomy surgery (removal of the thyroid). With all these extra cancers turning up, you would expect the rate of deaths from thyroid cancer to also increase (doctors can't cure every case they see) or maybe decrease (due to early detection) but the mortality from thyroid cancer barely changed over that time. It turned out that doctors were just diagnosing a lot more low-grade papillary cancers and treating them, often unnecessarily.

A 2015 study looking at rates of thyroid cancer from around the world noted that there has been a steady increase in thyroid cancer diagnosis rates (mainly papillary cancer) but mostly without a corresponding increase in death rates. Individual studies from many countries all show the same thing; one study concluded that this was 'not an epidemic of disease but rather an epidemic of diagnosis'.

The increased rates of thyroid cancer in all of these countries pale into insignificance compared to those in South Korea, where thyroid cancer has become the poster child for overdiagnosis. A screening program for many cancers began in 1999, and although thyroid cancer wasn't on the list, it could be tagged on for a few extra bucks and, well, why not?

A lot of patients got tested for thyroid cancer. That was good for the GPs who ordered the tests and who often did the ultrasound in their office. It was also good for the other people doing the ultrasounds and for people doing the more expensive tests – the MRIs and even pricier positron emission tomography (PET) scans. And it was good for the surgeons who got paid to take out thyroids, not to mention the hospitals that marketed the screening and got paid for the treatment.

Thyroid cancer rates increased 15-fold from 1993 to 2011, particularly taking off after the government ramped up cancer screening. Importantly, the rates of cancer varied from region to region, depending on how aggressive the screening was in each region. This means that the 'epidemic' wasn't a true underlying increase in thyroid cancers, but simply an increase in the number of cancers being detected through screening. In other words, screening was finding cancers that had previously gone undetected, many of which would have remained hidden and never done any harm.

The situation got so crazy that thyroid cancer became the number one cancer diagnosed in South Korea – 40 000 people each year were diagnosed, most of them in young people and disproportionately in young women. Thyroid cancer is nowhere near the most common cancer in other countries. As if getting a diagnosis of thyroid cancer wasn't bad enough, nearly all patients were treated with thyroidectomy – surgical removal of the whole thyroid gland. Apart from the complications of surgery itself, because they no longer have a thyroid, and we all need the thyroid hormone it produces to live, these people are on lifetime thyroid replacement pills. Other complications include vocal cord paralysis, affecting ability to speak, in 2 per cent of cases; and loss of the parathyroid hormones (from accidently removing the small parathyroid glands at the same time as removing the thyroid) in 11 per cent. The parathyroid hormones are essential for regulating calcium and bone strength; having them removed requires close monitoring and lifetime treatment.

This was always going to happen once they started looking for thyroid cancers. It has long been known that about a third of all people carry small thyroid cancers, most of which would never kill them or cause any problems at all. It has also long been known that if you look at the thyroids of dead people who didn't die of thyroid cancer, you're very likely to find thyroid cancers just sitting there that were undetected in life.

The people who had surgery largely had small relatively inactive tumours, many of which would have best been treated by just watching the patient and not removing it. Surgery for cancers less than 1 centimetre in diameter made up 14 per cent of all South Korean thyroid surgeries in 1995 but 56 per cent of all thyroid surgeries ten years later.

And what happened to the number of people dying from thyroid cancer each year? It stayed exactly the same. There was no epidemic of deadly cancers, and all the screening to detect 'early' cancers was a waste of time. So while the South Korean program was successful in diagnosing cancer, and the business around it boomed, it also led to tens of thousands of people being unnecessarily diagnosed with cancer each year, having their thyroid removed and sustaining the associated complications of that surgery. And yet the same number of people were dying from thyroid cancer each year. Only recently was the program finally wound down.

Cancer screening in Japanese children

Neuroblastoma is a severe form of cancer that occurs in young children. It arises from nerve cells, most commonly in and around the adrenal glands (just above the kidneys). In 1985, Japan initiated a mass screening program for all children at six months of age, screening more than 1 million children over the next two decades. The program was initiated after a study reported that a mass screening program for neuroblastoma in Kyoto had resulted in an increase in survival of neuroblastoma patients from 17 to 72 per cent. Observations from the outcomes of the screening program seemed to back this up – of about 1900 cases detected, more than 97 per cent were still alive at long-term follow-up. But after two trials performed in Germany and Canada showed no benefit, the program was re-evaluated. A Japanese committee concluded in 2003 that the testing had led to overdiagnosis and had not reduced mortality from the condition. Most of the cancers that had been detected had a favourable prognosis and didn't need to be found, while the mortality rate (which was unchanged) was due to the more deadly neuroblastomas that develop in older children and were never going to be detected by screening six-month-olds. The screening program was stopped in 2004.

Prostate cancer: to screen or not to screen?

Abnormally high levels of PSA in the blood may indicate the presence of prostate cancer but, like most things in medicine, it's not that straightforward. People without prostate cancer can have elevated levels of PSA too, and lots of men, more commonly as they get older, have prostate cancer. Like thyroid cancer, it's a very common finding in autopsies of men who never had a problem with prostate cancer during their lifetime.

PSA testing became very popular in the 1980s and 1990s and, as a result, lots more men were diagnosed with prostate cancer. A lot of those cancers were removed by surgery (prostatectomy) but roughly the same number of people were dying of prostate cancer each year. This means we weren't saving more lives by diagnosing more cancers. If we'd been identifying and treating more men with *harmful* prostate cancer earlier, we would have expected the number of deaths to decline. We now know that too many prostatectomies were being done. Surgeons are now a lot more selective about who they operate on. In fact, while in the decade up to 1992 the rate of prostatectomy surgery roughly doubled due to a rise in PSA testing, over the next three years it more than halved for men aged over 70.

The harms from prostatectomy are actually pretty significant, but even if those harms are accurately conveyed to the patient, it's hard to take them into consideration when you've been told you have cancer and someone is offering to remove it. Roughly 20 per cent of men will have problems with urination and/or sexual function after a prostatectomy. There are also many other potential general complications of surgery, such as blood loss, blood clots, pain and infection – and, of course, death.

In 2018, the US Preventive Services Task Force recommended against PSA screening in men aged 70 and over, and concluded that even for younger men the balance of benefits and harms is fairly even. A high-quality Cochrane review (see chapter 10) of prostate cancer screening was blunter. It found that prostate cancer screening does not save lives, harms are frequent, and overdiagnosis and overtreatment are common. It's telling as well that countries like Australia have no government-sponsored prostate cancer screening programs such as those in place for cervical, breast and bowel cancer.

Breast cancer screening: still hotly debated

It would be remiss of us not to mention one of the largest screening programs in the world: mammography for breast cancer. It leads to many cases being diagnosed, which sounds good, but nearly all the extra cases are mild cancers that may not have harmed the woman in her lifetime. In particular, the mildest form, called ductal cancer in situ (DCIS) or Stage 0 cancer, now makes up around a quarter of all cancers detected by screening. Previously it made up only 1 per cent of cancers. DCIS is almost entirely detected by mammography, does not necessarily progress to cancer, can regress without treatment, and potentially harmful treatments such as radiation treatment may not be helpful. The benefits of treating DCIS have not been compared to having no treatment (other than regular monitoring to make sure things have not changed), but some trials are currently underway. At the moment, just about everyone gets treated. Some women with multiple DCIS cancers or those in whom new ones are frequently found on annual mammograms, opt to have bilateral mastectomies so they can get off the merry-go-round, and who can blame them? They are constantly playing Russian roulette, not knowing if or when a DCIS might just progress to invasive cancer.

We do have good evidence on mammography screening programs. Large-scale randomised trials involving hundreds of thousands of women have been done comparing screening to usual care. In a high-quality review of those trials (from the Cochrane Collaboration; see chapter 10), the effect on breast-cancer-specific death – that is, deaths specifically *from* breast cancer – was marginally better in the women who had been randomised to receive the screening. But the review judged the use of disease-specific deaths to be unreliable and biased in favour of screening. The real test of screening programs designed to reduce death is the 'all-cause' overall death rate – that is, deaths from all causes. So how much less likely to die were the women who were screened? The death rate in the screened and unscreened groups was almost exactly the same. In fact, there were actually a few *more* deaths in the screening group after ten years.

The review found that many women who undergo screening will be diagnosed unnecessarily. Women who were screened were more likely to be told they had cancer and more likely to undergo biopsy, surgery and radiation treatment. But their chances of dying were the same as those of the women who didn't have screening mammography.

The benefits and risks of mammography are still hotly debated, but as you can see the benefits are not clear. Even if there are benefits (for example, some people may benefit from early detection of a less common, serious tumour), we have to balance these benefits against the real physical and psychological harms resulting from the much more common scenario of overdiagnosis and unnecessary treatment, including radiation and surgery. Many reviews and government recommendations have come out against screening for breast cancer. Yet screening remains commonplace, partly because it sounds like a good idea and partly because it is entrenched in our thinking and in medicine's business model.

Lung cancer screening: new kid on the block

Several countries around the world have started screening smokers or former smokers for lung cancer using low-dose CT scans (LDCT), which expose the person to less radiation than the older CT scans. A report prepared by Cancer Australia for the Australian Government in 2020 recommends a national rollout of regular screening for smokers and ex-smokers aged 50–74 years. This will cost hundreds of millions of dollars to provide. The report is based on evidence from seven randomised trials, which were summarised in a systematic review published in 2020. The report concludes that 12 000 lung cancer deaths would be prevented by screening, which sounds like a worthwhile benefit. Surprisingly for such a recent report, there's no mention whatsoever of the effect of screening on *overall* mortality.

The same systematic review provides this important missing information, however: it shows that there's no statistically significant or clinically important difference in overall deaths from screening when all seven studies are combined. The summary results are heavily influenced by the two largest studies, which contributed about 75 per cent of the pooled result. In one of those two studies, the difference in overall deaths between those screened and those not screened was 0.5 per cent in favour of screening, and in the other (the most recent study), the difference was 0.2 per cent in favour of *not* screening. Neither of these results were statistically significant, which basically means there was no difference between the groups at all.

The report does mention that the false-negative rate (where cancer is present but not detected) is up to 1.3 per cent, while the false-positive rate (where cancer is diagnosed, but not actually present) is, at best, 1.2 per cent. Based upon the most recent study, it also estimates an overdiagnosis rate of 8.9 per cent, meaning there's a risk that almost one in 11 people could receive a diagnosis that doesn't help them.

It's quite possible that screening for lung cancer in high-risk people (as proposed in the report) will save lives. But the best evidence we have does not support that conclusion, and the number of people who will be unnecessarily diagnosed and treated (commonly with surgery) in such a national program will be high.

Ovarian cancer screening: waiting in the wings

A large-scale randomised study (involving more than 200 000 women) comparing two types of ovarian cancer screening to no screening was reported in the *Lancet* in 2021. After following patients for more than 15 years, the researchers found that the incidence of tubal or ovarian cancer, and the death rate from these cancers, was the same in all three groups (the two screening groups and the no screening group).

In a previous publication of the same study published five years earlier, the authors (despite also showing no clear advantage to screening) were optimistic, stating 'the results suggested that an unequivocally significant difference in mortality might emerge after longer follow-up'.

In both studies, the authors refer to the effect on 'mortality', but they are referring to 'disease-specific mortality', not overall mortality. In fact, no reference is made to overall mortality, and no results pertaining to overall (all-cause) mortality are provided in the manuscripts or supplementary material, despite this being necessary and easy to measure. To us, not reporting the difference in 'actual' mortality (i.e. the number of people who died in each group, regardless of the cause) is not providing us with the most important information.

The complication rate in the screened group was higher than in the unscreened group, and many women who were screened had surgery to remove tumours that were later found to be benign. Even though we don't know the effect of screening on overall mortality, it appears that ovarian cancer screening provides no benefit but some harm.

The bottom line on population screening

The simplistic notion of screening everyone for disease to save lives has appeal, but it just doesn't stack up. A 2016 review concluded that although the results of cancer screening were often biased in favour of screening, the bottom line was that screening often didn't change the chance of people dying.

Even if a person were to die at exactly the same time in their life from a cancer that was identified by screening compared to one that wasn't, screening would still come out looking better. This is because of something called lead-time bias. Let's say screening detects the cancer at age 60, and the patient dies at age 80. And let's say that if they hadn't had screening, the cancer would have been picked up at age 70 and they still would have died at age 80. The 'survival time' with cancer would be 20 years with screening and only ten years without screening, so screening would have doubled the survival time with cancer, but without providing one extra day of life for the patient – and they would have known they had cancer for ten years longer. This is how screening programs can be made to look effective, despite offering no benefit. They result in the patient having to live longer with the knowledge they have cancer.

Health recommendations, when applied on such a large scale and at such a cost to society, deserve to be properly thought through and not accepted on good intentions alone. What if, for example, in the process of trying to prevent a disease (not just cancer) we incorrectly label many people with that disease, worrying those people unnecessarily and subjecting them to further tests, such as biopsies and dangerous treatments? And in the process, what if those we correctly identify with the disease are left stranded because there's no good treatment for them? Or what if the treatment for established disease is simple, effective and cheap? Is it then worth the extra effort of subjecting all non-diseased people to screening? We're too quick to assume that ideas that sound good and are well intentioned are correct, instead of adopting a more objective, sceptical attitude and waiting for evidence that shows whether these ideas are right.

In 1968, the WHO produced a list of ten criteria that need to be satisfied to ensure a screening program is effective. These include such things as the need to minimise the risks of screening and determine the costs. But two crucial criteria are often at the centre of arguments about current screening programs:

- The overall benefits of screening should outweigh the harm.
- There should be scientific evidence that the screening program is effective.

Many current screening programs don't satisfy these criteria, providing no significant health improvement for individual patients or communities. And many of those same programs are still actively promoted, particularly by those who are heavily invested in the screening industry.

The WHO criteria were updated in 2008 to include consideration of genetic screening. Note was again made of the ever-widening gap between what's technologically possible and the desire to introduce or expand screening programs before the necessary safeguards and regulations are in place. The updated criteria place greater emphasis on informed choice, respect for autonomy, equity of access, and evidence to ensure the intended aims are being met.

The role of the media

The media often report newsworthy claims without substantiating their scientific merit. Headlines and reports portray 'breakthroughs' and miracle cures, tending to emphasise or exaggerate the potential benefits of any new treatments while minimising or ignoring the harms. But these good news stories aren't balanced by stories showing when popular treatments have been proven ineffective.

The media like to focus on stories about life-saving treatments whose effectiveness can't be proven. Because trained journalists often feel the need to present a 'balanced' case, they will counter-balance well-supported scientific evidence with an opposing opinion that has no basis in fact.

We have both been frustrated when our own research has been reported in this way. For example, when trying to promote research showing that spinal surgery for back pain may not be helpful and may make people worse, journalists will tend to 'balance' the article by including the personal story of a patient who improved after surgery, or interviewing a surgeon who disagrees. The problem with journalistic 'bothsidesism' is that it leaves the consumer thinking either that the truth lies somewhere between the two opposing opinions, or that we don't know the real answer. The common possibility that one view is correct and the other view wrong is rarely portrayed or considered.

Despite this desire for balance, the media often report imbalanced stories. For example, stories about screening will include people who have been 'saved' by screening but not the people who make the decision not to be screened, or who were harmed by screening. The media also have a preference for lower-quality observational studies over randomised trials (possibly because they are easier to understand), tend not to investigate and disclose conflicts of interest (from the doctor or the media organisation, which is benefiting from advertorials), and often use biased or non-expert commentators. The changing media environment has led to more of this 'junk-food news'.

* * *

Doctors are failing to avoid the trap of overtreatment. In their desire to detect and treat, they frequently overtreat, often resulting in no benefit and in net harm. Furthermore, the evidence for this is often not sought or is suppressed. Instead, doctors rely on simplistic notions that more is better, and continue to overestimate the benefits and underestimate the harms of their actions.

4

Warmth and sympathy

Hippocratic Oath: I will remember that there is art to medicine as well as science, and that warmth, sympathy, and understanding may outweigh the surgeon's knife or the chemist's drug.

'Cure sometimes, treat often, comfort always'
– attributed to Hippocrates

'Caring without science is well-intentioned kindness, but not medicine. On the other hand, science without caring empties medicine of healing and negates the great potential of an ancient profession. The two complement and are essential to the art of doctoring.'
– Bernard Lown, US cardiologist, *The Lost Art of Healing*

The Mid Staffordshire scandal, considered one of the worst hospital scandals of recent times, highlights what happens when empathy is removed from care. Around 2005–08, the main hospital serving the Mid Staffordshire region of England was the subject of many complaints from patients and their relatives due to poor standards of care. The complaints included such things as patients drinking out of vases because their water was left out of reach, and being left in their own excrement for lengthy periods.

The complaints initially led to local inquiries, which found that the hospital was performing satisfactorily, at least according to the standards used to measure hospital performance. No systemic

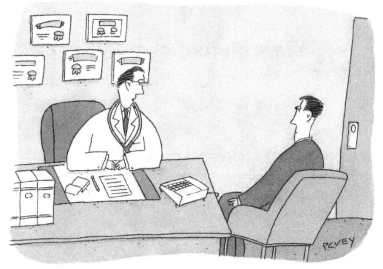

"There's no easy way I can tell you this, so I'm sending you to someone who can."

failures were noted. A high death rate was reported, but nothing untoward in the day-to-day standards used to measure hospital performance. The hospital itself initially put the high number of deaths down to 'coding errors'.

But the complaints about the hospital related to a lack of empathy rather than specifics or technicalities of medical care. Leaving water out of reach, not assisting helpless patients with toileting and feeding, and not providing privacy showed that patients weren't treated with the respect and dignity they should expect from carers with the necessary empathy and compassion.

Later inquiries showed the problems to be widespread across the hospital, and to extend beyond the complaints listed above, including the loss of hundreds of lives due to poor care or lack of care. In short, although the system was ticking boxes for standards, it wasn't working for the patients. It was working for itself – coming in on budget and managing, for the time being anyway, negative perceptions.

The Mid Staffordshire disaster could be seen as arising from a system that lacked empathy. A major contributing factor was that care wasn't patient-focused but instead focused on the *processes* of care.

At the core of the 'art' of medicine is compassion, a crucial factor in any communication between doctor and patient. Lack of compassion is one of the most common reasons behind healthcare complaints and lawsuits against doctors. Patients will forgive a lot if they feel that they have been valued, respected, understood and genuinely cared for in line with their best interests. But there are many more reasons for compassion to be front and centre in any doctor–patient interaction.

Is the 'art' of medicine quantifiable?

Communicating with patients with empathy and compassion has been shown to be associated with better health outcomes, fewer doctor visits and less medication. But the evidence for benefits arising from being more compassionate is not widely known and the area isn't widely studied, partly because it's hard to study or to measure precisely. We know that patients are more satisfied with their medical treatment when doctors show them dignity and respect. Patients also have a basic expectation that they will be treated in this way.

People treated with empathy are more likely to be satisfied with their overall care and to stick to their treatments. Greater empathy has been shown, for example, to improve vaccination levels and diabetes management. This shows that interpersonal factors such as empathy and compassion can magnify or increase the benefit of the specific treatments given. Interpersonal factors can also explain much of the benefit of treatments that have no specific inherent benefit of their own. In one study, patients with irritable bowel syndrome (IBS) were given placebo acupuncture, but some of them had the treatment delivered by a warm, empathic and confident practitioner. The group given the treatment *plus* these positive interpersonal factors showed significantly greater improvement.

Empathy also plays a role in reducing patient anxiety and stress, and in generating trust between patient and doctor. These factors are helpful for the process of shared decision-making. This works from both sides: the doctor can better tailor the content and delivery of information if they understand the concerns and fears of the patient; and if the patient trusts and understands their doctor, they are less stressed, and find the decision-making process more comfortable and satisfying.

A review of all randomised studies that have investigated this techniques showed that, compared to usual care, empathy or positive messaging were consistently associated with improved health outcomes, including pain, anxiety, distress, satisfaction, quality of life and even specific disease symptoms such as those from IBS.

The doctor also benefits from taking a more empathetic approach to patient care. Doctors who show greater empathy during patient interactions have greater professional quality of life and job satisfaction. They are also less likely to suffer from burnout and to have complaints made against them.

Why don't doctors use empathy more?

There are several reasons. Firstly, the problem is part of the very mechanistic, 'reductionist' approach in medicine that stems from the disease–illness paradigm, whereby diseases are seen as strictly the results of single, physically identifiable causes. This distils complaints down to their essence, a specific diagnosis, and focuses on the delivery of a specific treatment targeting that specific diagnosis. Medical training emphasises this way of thinking over the non-specific, interpersonal aspects of care, such as making the patient feel valued, assuring them if their fears are ill founded, increasing their understanding and addressing their anxieties.

While empathy and compassion *are* taught in medical school, the effectiveness of this training varies, and the amount of time devoted to it and the emphasis placed upon it also vary. Yet there is evidence that it is possible to teach these skills. A systematic review of curricula for empathy and compassion training in medical education, which included 52 studies involving well over 5000 medical students, found that several behaviours can be taught that improve patient perception of a doctor's empathy and compassion. A common feature in these behaviours is a focus on being fully present, listening and being aware of the patient's emotional state. Important learned behaviours that improve empathy and compassion include sitting rather than standing during the consultation, detecting and responding to patients' non-verbal cues of emotion and to opportunities for compassion, using eye contact and other non-verbal ways of communicating caring, and using words that acknowledge, validate and support the patient.

Another argument is that medicine focuses too much on technological solutions. But technology has created other barriers to an empathic approach. Modern medical imaging replaces the physical contact from a doctor's examination, and electronic monitoring replaces physical contact from nurses (e.g. taking a pulse or temperature). Physical contact is an important part of empathy and communication, but it's also an important part of medical care. The act of holding a hand has alone been shown to help with pain and stress levels.

Another factor is the lack of time to provide empathy and the lack of incentives to do so. This is part of the problem with current business models for medicine – because they are focused on time-based processes, they don't incentivise interpersonal factors in care. In other words, they concentrate on maximising turnover.

No business model in medicine encourages a doctor to take more time listening to a patient and to be more compassionate. In fact, most models discourage these aspects of care. The devaluing of compassion has left us with fewer options for treatment, fuelling the bias towards doing *something* over doing *nothing*. When specific tests and treatments are the only tools to rely on, that's what will be used, even in cases where assurance and compassion are all that's required.

Medicine as a business

Despite being treated as a business, medicine doesn't fit a business or free-market model. A free market implies choice, and the option not to enter the marketplace at all. Choice sounds fine, but when an illness is unexpected, which is usually the case, there's rarely the time or opportunity to exercise choice in providers or to shop around for better deals, and there's basically no choice to opt out.

If we see medical care as a right, it should be made available. Yet given the costs of care, or even of insurance, many people can't afford it. So if healthcare is a right, and many, including the United Nations, believe it is, it's up to governments, or very large private donors, to ensure that it's supplied to all who need it.

One of the biggest barriers to the provision of health care is its cost, but why is it so expensive? Firstly, medicine doesn't follow simple economic rules, like that of supply and demand. Instead of the supply of doctors satisfying the demand for healthcare, doctors create the demand. If you have a problem with long waiting lists for surgery, supplying more surgeons will only get you more waiting lists of a similar size. Particularly in a fee-for-service setting, more doctors means more tests and treatments as they work to fill the time available to them by filling operating lists, requesting tests, writing prescriptions, and finding more and more things to treat. Why does their work expand to fill the time available? Because medicine is a business, and that's how everybody in it makes money. More medical care means more money for everyone involved.

The profit motive is not limited to the doctors. For all the players in the delivery of medical care: the hospital owners, drug companies, drug dispensers, implant and device manufacturers, sales reps and everyone else who works in the system, more care is better, and higher prices are better.

If we make medicine a business, we're seeking profit. Those involved will charge whatever the market will bear and, as in any business, turnover is key. Simply put, the best business model for medicine is one where as much medicine is done as possible, at the highest possible prices. There are several consequences to this. Firstly, many patients will be priced out of the care they need, and secondly, many will be given care that isn't needed, at prices that aren't justified. The business of medicine relies on maximising the number of sick people to treat. A healthy community is bad for business.

Beyond the level of individual patient care and how it has been monetised lies another level of business: the 'really big' business of drug companies. The interests of hospital owners and insurers are clear, and they will always seek to have some control over the medical system in order to favour their profits. Drug companies are in another league. As some of the largest companies in the world, their power to tilt the playing field to their advantage is huge, and their business model is to treat as many people with as many drugs as possible at the greatest cost. While drug effectiveness is part of that model, so is *perception* of effectiveness. To this end, drug companies can bury research that isn't favourable to their product, and they can lobby governments to change the rules regarding the level of proof of effectiveness required to market the drugs.

In the United States in particular, the rules governing proof of effectiveness for new drugs before approval have been relaxed. Rules regarding patent extensions, the use of generic drugs, and drug pricing have favoured big drug companies. It may be argued that this isn't necessarily done in direct response to massive lobbying and donations from drug companies, but one could also argue that if lobbying and political donations weren't a good return on investment, responsible companies wouldn't bother with them.

A recent example of questionable drug approval, and the surrounding positive spin regarding effectiveness, is the expensive Alzheimer's drug aducanumab (listed price US$56 000 per year). It received fast-track approval by the FDA despite its own scientific advisory panel previously rejecting it on the basis that the evidence for effectiveness was not convincing. While the studies had found that the drug can reduce the amount of beta-amyloid plaque in the brain, they did not show it reduces cognitive decline.

The FDA's reversal of its earlier decision was made on the basis of a reanalysis of the previous trials that focused on a small subgroup of people who might benefit from taking high doses of the drug. The approval was conditional on the company conducting another study to prove that this is the case. Yet in the meantime there is no way of knowing who this subgroup might be and if others might be harmed. Aducanumab can cause severe adverse effects including confusion, and bleeding and swelling of the brain.

The drug company has touted the approval as a 'win for patients'. According to *The Age* newspaper, the Australian Health Minister, Greg Hunt, has indicated he would make it available on the pharmaceutical benefits scheme in Australia if it is approved by the Therapeutic Goods Administration (the Australian equivalent of the FDA). He said, 'It's a sign of hope, I met with the company [Biogen] a few years ago when they were developing it'.

Even at the level of the patient, the problem wouldn't be so bad without information asymmetry, meaning the patient doesn't have the information available to question or properly contribute to the decision-making process. Information asymmetry (between doctors and patients or insurers and patients) opens the door for exploitation. This is yet another reason to have well-informed patients.

Choosing words carefully

The power of language to influence people's opinions and decisions is well known, and it's no different in the important interaction between doctors and their patients. This part of the art of medicine can be used to raise, or lower, the level of a patient's fear regarding a diagnosis, forcing them either to find a way to allay the fear or mitigate the risk. The practitioner then offers the treatment as the solution, and here again the use of language can bias the patient's interpretation of the risks and benefits, making the treatment appear more acceptable.

If it were a con, the diagnosis would be the set-up and the treatment would be the pay-off. In our current, procedure-focused, fee-for-service system, the treatment really is the pay-off. Doctors who perform procedures earn a lot more from doing things to patients (procedures) than from not doing them. It's no coincidence that being a surgeon is the highest paid job in Australia.

Doctors can quite easily talk up a patient's fear from a diagnosis. To a patient with narrowed coronary arteries, they might say, 'You have a time-bomb in your chest', or to a patient with normal degenerative changes in the spine, 'There are multiple ruptured discs in your spine' or 'It's a mess'. Language can be used to create or inflate the patient's uncertainty – 'It could go either way' or 'We just don't know' – thus leading the patient towards the nearest certainty: the treatment.

More insidious is what *isn't* said. Just seeing the reports of an angiogram or MRI can be a frightening experience. The report might say something like: 'a 50 per cent narrowing of the left main coronary artery' or 'multiple levels of disc degeneration'. Unless their doctor clearly indicates the often-benign significance of these findings, patients will fear the worst. Studies have shown that the use of technical medical terms in scan results can increase patient anxiety and make them perceive their condition as more severe, encouraging a preference for more invasive care and further testing. One study found that use of clearer and less 'emotive' language to describe harmless changes in upper-limb MRI reports reduced patient worry.

In presenting the treatment options, doctors tend to see their treatments as better and less harmful than they really are, so the language they use may seem appropriate to them. But language can have a strong effect. An orthopaedic surgeon can easily sell surgery to operate on a broken bone even if the evidence for surgery is unclear, by giving the patient a choice between surgery to 'fix' the fracture or leaving it alone. The surgeon uses the word 'fix' in a surgical context, meaning to stabilise or hold fast using screws and plates, like fixing (or fastening) a shelf to a wall. But the patient may well interpret the word fix as meaning to 'repair' or 'make good'. The patient may also interpret 'leaving it alone' in a negative light, as 'neglect', whereas the surgeon simply means not operating, perhaps by applying a sling, bandage or plaster. And if the surgeon doesn't mention that the likelihood of healing and good function is similar for both treatments, the patient will think that surgery is the superior option.

Again, what isn't said is important. Saying that a stent will 'unblock' an artery doesn't tell the patient whether this is in their best interests; without this explanation, it is *implied* that the unblocking procedure is a good thing and better than not unblocking it. Creating urgency also pushes patients towards treatment: 'Fortunately, there's a slot in tomorrow's schedule so we can get this done quickly'.

A doctor's words can also be directly harmful. Even though it's appropriate to inform patients of the possible side effects of drugs, studies have shown that merely making patients aware of the side effects makes them more likely to complain of experiencing them. This may be because of heightened awareness and expectations. The same occurs with symptoms: if the doctor tells a patient they will continue to have symptoms without treatment, they will be more likely to complain of those symptoms in the future; it can become a self-fulfilling prophecy. Patients can also take doctors' words literally. One patient who had had a heart attack was told on discharge from hospital that he was 'all fixed'. He then failed to turn up for the rehabilitation program that was organised for him because he didn't see the need – he was all fixed. These sorts of misunderstandings happen all the time.

Doctors also use the persuasive art of rhetoric to convey positive messages about their treatment. Saying that the proposed treatment is 'the latest', 'what everybody's doing now', 'targets your disease specifically', or 'very safe now' says nothing of its effectiveness or, for that matter, its actual safety. And saying 'There's now quite a lot of research on this treatment' doesn't tell the patient whether that research is favourable, but does make them think it is. Doctors, like salespeople, spend a lot of time talking to people and guiding their decision-making. With practice, it becomes easy to project your own wishes onto the patient.

The rhetoric of medicine is also used in health advertising and in programs aimed at medicalising normal people: 'Can you afford to not know? Come in for a whole-body scan today, to give you peace of mind'. Even the use of scientific terms is a form of rhetoric. It can impress the patient and appeal to their beliefs that things that sound scientific are more likely to be reliable and true. All professions use their own complex terms in this way – to separate themselves from and intimidate those outside the profession, and to give the appearance of greater knowledge. We all encounter this problem when talking to professions outside our own – for example, IT, law and accountancy.

Doctors can also use language in a positive way, of course – by explaining that the changes on an MRI are normal for people the patients' age, unrelated to the presence of symptoms, that the outlook is good, and that simple non-operative treatment is preferred and likely to result in improvement. This reassures the patient and reduces their stress levels. If the doctor shows a genuine concern and willingness to work in the patient's best interests while delivering this message, it helps both the patient and the doctor.

Mismatched doctor–patient communication

The bias towards acting instead of holding back and simply listening or assuring someone has other drivers. There's a known mismatch between what doctors would accept for themselves and what they do for their patients. Studies have shown that in terminal care, for example, both patients and doctors would prefer less aggressive care at the end of life and would rather die comfortably than undergo intensive treatments aimed at extending life. But instead, aggressive care becomes the default recommended by doctors.

We also know there's a mismatch between what patients want and what doctors think they want. Patients seek care for many different reasons. They might seek diagnostic clarification, reassurance, legitimation of their symptoms, a 'cure' for their complaints or symptomatic relief. They might sometimes just wish to express distress, frustration or anger. Because the appropriate responses to these reasons vary, it's essential that doctors clarify *why* the patient is there. Yet evidence suggests that there are often communication misunderstandings, and patients may not voice all their agenda items, both of which lead to poorer outcomes. For example, patients may not voice their worries about the possible diagnosis and what the future holds, what's wrong with them, side effects, *not* wanting a prescription and so on.

Doctors and other health professionals often overestimate their communication skills. A series of studies in emergency departments revealed the complexity of the interactions that unfold between doctors and patients. One Australian study followed the patient's journey from the time they arrived in the emergency department to the moment a decision was made about whether they needed to stay in hospital for treatment or could go home. A researcher sat quietly in the corner of the room observing and recording all interactions that took place between the patient and the medical team. In many instances it took the doctor a long time to figure out the true reason for the visit. This was often because there was a mismatch between what the patient wanted to say or was trying to say and what the doctor wanted to know.

Typically, the doctor initiated the exchange by asking very specific medically oriented questions. In one instance the doctors and nurses asked 145 questions of an elderly woman whose first language wasn't English before finally landing on what prompted her visit. On the other hand, patients asked very few questions and were rarely given the opportunity to deviate from the question–answer format. This restricted exploration of the patients' main reasons for visiting and limited the doctors' chances to respond to the patients' concerns and need for information.

Other studies have explored the mismatch in the experience of the doctor–patient consultation by interviewing both the doctor and the patient after a consultation ('paired interviews'). These studies have shed light on the contrasts between the mindset of patients and that of the doctors. In one study that explored paired interviews of patients with chronic back pain, notable mismatches were found between the patient and the doctor in how the problem was perceived. The patient had a very medical or biomechanical model of their problem and wanted a definitive diagnosis, while the doctor had a more biopsychosocial model of illness. Treatment expectations also varied, the patient being focused on the goal of reducing pain, and the doctors on improving function. Identifying and addressing such significant differences in thinking seems crucial for doctors to build empathic relationships with patients and optimising care.

Another communication problem between doctors and patients

is information asymmetry, where the doctor and patient have insufficient information about each other's views. This contributes to the 'moral hazard', an economics theme that refers to a situation where the person taking the risk is protected because someone else will bear the cost. In medicine, it's the difference in potential harm between the person making the decision (largely, the doctor) and the person bearing the potential harm (the patient). In other words, a doctor may be more likely to recommend a risky procedure because they won't be suffering the harm if it occurs. It explains why, for example, so many orthopaedic surgeons put up with their arthritic knee, but are happy to recommend knee replacement surgery to their patients with similar symptoms. This distortion of decision-making is partly due to a lack of communication, but also a lack of empathy.

Shared decision-making

The natural result of using empathy and including the patient's perspective is that the decision-making process about care truly is shared between a well-informed patient and their doctor or other healthcare professional. Shared decision-making is an often-stated goal, but the execution sometimes falls short. Studies have shown that increasing patient education and involvement in the decision-making process yields such benefits as improved patient satisfaction with their decisions and less indecision. It results in better, more complete and more precise understanding of the risks and benefits of different care options. Perhaps most importantly, shared decision-making often leads to different decisions being made, sometimes avoiding treatments initially recommended by doctors.

The most comprehensive review of doctors using decision aids (tools to provide patients with better information) to support shared decision-making showed that patients involved in this process were less likely to choose low-value or ineffective treatments, including some forms of elective surgery, prostate cancer screening and cardiac stress testing. The icing on the cake is that patients were *more* likely to choose some high-value care options, such as hepatitis vaccinations and the use of medication for uncontrolled diabetes.

Some experts have argued against the concept and use of shared decision-making, saying that patients don't care about the numbers, might get confused by the probabilities, and will trust the doctor's decision. This may be true, but there's sufficient evidence to say we shouldn't necessarily trust the doctor with those decisions. They often have a biased view of the benefits and harms, they don't necessarily recommend what they would want for themselves, and they're not the ones taking the risk. It's a bit like leaving all your investments in the hands of an adviser. If you simply go with their recommendations, you won't be happy if it all goes wrong, but if you had a part in the decision-making, you might be more comfortable with the outcome, however bad.

Some argue against shared decision-making on the basis of insufficient time. But this is time well spent and doesn't take much longer than not using it.

The failure of legal control of medical harm

Poor communication is one of the main reasons for medical malpractice suits, but the legal control of medical harm is centred around negligence, and negligence is only one small contributing factor to medical harm. Much medical harm comes from *unnecessary* medical care rather than negligent or poorly conducted care, and unnecessary care is rarely litigated.

Lawyers claim that the laws around medical malpractice keep medical practice in check and serve to minimise bad practice. Others would say that the medical malpractice system is centred on maximising financial returns to clients and lawyers (on one side) and avoidance of litigation (on the other) rather than improved quality of care, and thus fails to improve medical care. We agree with this second view, at least partly because the malpractice system has been around for a long time without reducing medical harm. Despite constant fear of litigation, doctors still harm people and provide unnecessary care, often because of the very fear of litigation.

In 'defensive medicine', doctors change their practice to decrease their risk of being sued, normally by requesting too many tests, prescribing more treatments and doing more procedures than is necessary. The result is overtesting, overdiagnosis and overtreatment. And the problem is real. Studies have shown that doctors admit to the practice, and there's some evidence that it's associated with fewer malpractice claims. In other words, the legal system can increase the harms of medicine (any unnecessary test or treatment still carries harms), harms that aren't addressed by the system that created them. For example, a patient who has complications from surgery may sue the surgeon, but they will rarely sue the doctor who ordered the unnecessary scan that led to the unnecessary surgery. They will also focus on the care received during the surgery and the technical aspects of the procedure, not on whether the surgery was needed in the first place. It's highly unusual for a doctor to be sued for unnecessary treatment.

Is defensive medicine the price we pay to reduce errors? Medical negligence laws are based on 'deterrence theory' – deterring the errors that lead to lawsuits. Unfortunately, the evidence does not support any reduction in errors due to negligence claims, only an increase in defensive medicine. Medical negligence laws only deter doctors from getting sued, not from making errors.

We're not saying that bad practice doesn't exist. There are examples of doctors whose registration has been revoked for poor practice, but these are rare and often this happens as a result of deliberate actions. Most lawsuits are against the 'average' doctor, and they're not correlated with the quality of their practice.

Lawsuits against doctors start with an aggrieved patient. The likelihood of action against a doctor is closely related to the communication between the patient and the doctor. A patient who has been sufficiently heard by a doctor who has shown empathy, compassion and a genuine concern and desire to help them, will forgive many technical errors or complications and will be less likely to feel aggrieved. Many doctors who make less than optimal clinical decisions never get sued because their patients are satisfied with their care. Conversely, there are excellent doctors who, when an unavoidable complication occurs, get sued due to their poor bedside manner.

Communication content and style are particularly important when a complication or bad outcome occurs. Patients need to be informed of the problem, but the doctor also needs to show that they genuinely regret the problem, openly explain how and why it occurred, and explain how they will address it. Concealment or avoidance of responsibility after poor outcomes is a major cause of legal action.

But patients don't just claim 'poor communication' when suing their doctors. They are suing because they feel as if they weren't well treated. This leads us to the next problem: the definition of poor treatment. Often, a poor outcome is taken as evidence of poor treatment. But poor outcomes are common after medical treatment and, on their own, are not a case for legal action. The doctor not warning that the treatment might not work or that there could be complications or side effects signifies poor communication. But the mere presence of a poor outcome, such as an infection from surgery, an unexpected drug reaction or failure to improve, doesn't indicate poor treatment.

When a patient feels poorly treated, it's often because they feel *under*treated, and the complaint then focuses on why a treatment or test *wasn't* given. When patients *are* treated, the obvious question is never raised: was the test and/or treatment necessary in the first place? There is an inherent bias that treating is better than not treating regardless of the effectiveness of the treatment. An untreated patient feels they haven't been 'given the chance' the treatment would have provided, even when the probability of benefit from the treatment was negligible and the risks sizeable.

These problems all indicate that we need to take into account the patient's perspective in designing treatment solutions. We need to respect the patient's wishes and harness their capabilities, as well as those of their families and of society. Fortunately, patients are being involved more and more in medical care in general, not only through their inclusion in shared decision-making about their health and health care. Patients and consumers are also becoming more involved in doing the research.

Several frameworks now support patient and public involvement (PPI) in research, and increasingly this is being made a specific requirement for research funding. Involving people who have lived experience of the condition under study can improve the relevance and value of the research, improve recruitment and retention of study participants, and improve dissemination of the findings to the public. Partnering with patients and the public can also identify the most important questions as well as the most important outcomes to measure. The patient perspective can also benefit researchers by influencing their views on the research perspective.

* * *

Involving the public and patients in all aspects of health care, from designing and conducting research to making individual treatment decisions, leads to more appropriate and cost-effective health care, and better health outcomes. In the clinic it's up to doctors to encourage the patient to be involved, to listen and understand their values and perspective, and to empathise with them.

5

I know not

Hippocratic Oath: I will not be ashamed to say 'I know not',
nor will I fail to call in my colleagues when the skills of another
are needed for a patient's recovery.

'To do nothing is also a good remedy'
– attributed to Hippocrates

'In respect to evidence of curative processes … no one
knows in disease what is the simple result of nothing
being done, as a standard with which to compare'
– Charles Darwin

Why are doctors so reluctant to say 'I know not' when diagnosing and treating patients? This may occur in situations where doctors don't know or can't find the diagnosis and perhaps shouldn't even pursue a diagnosis, and when doctors don't have an effective treatment but feel the need to act, to do something rather than do nothing.

The use of the word 'ashamed' in this pledge of the Oath is important to our understanding of why doctors are reluctant to say 'I know not' and why they treat too much. Shame is a complex but powerful emotion, and one that doctors are reluctant to acknowledge. Uncoupling shame from saying 'I know not' is possible, once we understand why doctors feel ashamed to do so.

The key word here is 'failure'. To feel shame, you must consider it the result of a failure. People come to doctors for answers, and failure to answer their questions appears, well, like failure, and that causes the shame. Doctors need to stop seeing a failure to diagnose or treat as failing the *patient* or failing to provide *care*.

The repetitive strain injury epidemic

Repetitive strain (or stress) injury (RSI) arose as a diagnosis in the 1980s and was particularly prevalent in Australia. It was defined by a collection of symptoms, usually wrist, arm and hand pain. Unlike wrist and forearm conditions such as arthritis and tendinitis that have very specific symptoms and signs, for RSI there were no specific abnormalities that the doctor could find on examination, other than that the patient experienced pain when touched in the areas that were painful, and sometimes had muscle wasting due to lack of use of the arm and hand. It wasn't a disease with an identifiable cause. There was no physical evidence of stress or strain and, despite the name, RSI wasn't clearly correlated with repetitive strain or use.

RSI became common among people working in certain buildings and certain companies, and this distribution suggested it was more like something contagious (spreading by direct contact) than something with a mechanical cause. It usually started with one person in a workplace developing the syndrome and then being off work due to the 'injury', usually under workers' compensation insurance. Before long, other people in the same workplace were complaining of the same symptoms.

RSI reached an epidemic scale, particularly in Canberra and Sydney. At the time, it was attributed to the introduction of the computer keyboard, which replaced the typewriter in the 1980s. As computers allowed faster keystrokes than a typewriter, it was felt that the increased typing speed caused an injury to the structures in the hand and wrist. It was a good example of something that 'made sense' at a superficial level and was therefore assumed to be true.

RSI was similar to other occupational conditions, and subject to the same influences from stakeholders – unions, employers, insurers, lawyers, government, social workers, occupational therapists, physiotherapists and doctors. Similar types of illnesses had arisen in the past when technology changed. There was 'writer's cramp' when the steel nib was introduced, and 'telegrapher's cramp' when the telegraph was introduced. Like RSI, these illnesses were largely confined to groups of workers, usually in one building or company.

Initially, because it was thought to arise from work, employers were blamed for injuring their workers and were subjected to fines from regulators and lawsuits from patients. People with the condition were considered to be victims, often recognisable by the splints they wore, and there was considerable empathy for them. Eventually, however, the concentration of cases in clusters led to alternative theories about the cause. Rather than an overuse injury, psychosocial factors including a contagious fear of disease and bad employer–employee relations were implicated.

After several years, it was decided that there was no physical cause or any correlation with workplace conditions. Compensation for the condition was withdrawn, patients were no longer sick-listed, and lawsuits failed. After being treated as hapless victims of unsafe working environments, patients with RSI were now considered to be malingerers trying to milk the system, which was also wrong.

How did it spread if it wasn't physical? The answer is in the *way* it spread, by human contact or, to be more specific, human interaction. Someone had some wrist pain, which is common. Then they got worried about it, possibly exacerbated by a work-place dispute and/or stress. Other workers saw this and thought it might happen to them, which heightened their awareness of any possible wrist pain. The situation wasn't helped by the well-intentioned actions of the unions, which produced a publication called *The Sufferer's Handbook*; or the media, with headlines like 'Hi-tech epidemic: victims of a bright new technology that maims'.

The doctors' role wasn't helpful either. They're the ones who medicalised it by naming it and attributing it to the best explanation they could find at the time, which was, of course, a physical one. They also did the tests and biopsies and ordered the treatments (rest, splinting, medication), all of which reinforced the belief among the workers that they had a serious physical condition.

Fittingly, RSI was later described as an iatrogenic epidemic, meaning the epidemic was caused by doctors; by treating it as a medical condition, it became one. Although occupational conditions such as RSI have complex origins, the role of the doctors in making it worse, by medicalising, testing and treating, and basically fitting it into their disease–illness paradigm, is clear. The RSI epidemic in Australia was followed by a similar epidemic of 'cumulative trauma disorder' (CTD) in North America. While the epidemics have passed in terms of the sheer numbers of cases, both terms, RSI and CTD, are still used today to refer to a range of work-related upper-limb complaints, such as forearm, wrist and hand pain that have no other identifiable cause.

Would RSI have 'spread' if people complaining of wrist pain had been assured that their pain wasn't due to injury, and not given a label, treated and made to worry? Would it have become an epidemic if the doctors had just said 'I know not'? *

What exactly do patients want when they see a doctor, and what do they need? The two main types of questions doctors may answer are diagnostic and therapeutic. Diagnostic questions are to do with making a diagnosis and understanding the cause of a person's complaint. Therapeutic questions relate to treatment. The problem is that the patient seeking the answers may, in some circumstances, be better off without a diagnosis or treatment, and they may not be seeking either. They may just be seeking reassurance that their pain is normal.

As the RSI example illustrates, doctors' well-intentioned desire to diagnose doesn't necessarily lead to improved health. Some of the difficulties arise because we're trying to diagnose medical conditions or abnormalities that should be considered a normal part of life. Examples include some types of depression, fatigue, grief, and many of the changes that accompany ageing. Ill-defined symptoms such as headaches, general aches and pains, and other abnormal sensations such as dizziness, brain fog, stomach cramps and pins and needles, are also a normal part of life and don't necessarily benefit from a specific diagnosis.

Do predicaments of life benefit from diagnosis?

Labelling predicaments that are arguably a part of normal life is called 'medicalisation', which means bringing them into the medical domain. While this often occurs with good intentions, many conditions may be better off being left where they were, among the predicaments of life. Medicalisation favours the doctors: they get to control what happens and to dictate the policies, write the medical certificates, do the research, order the tests and provide the treatments for the new conditions they define. Doctors get to decide which difficulties and behaviours are 'pathological' and which aren't. Homosexuality, for example, was once considered pathological by the medical community.

In the past, some conditions, rather than being medicalised, were labelled and dealt with through religious or legal processes. 'Deviations' from normal, such as epilepsy, were labelled as sins by the church and managed in inhumane and harmful ways, with attempts to cast out the devil. Many people with mental health issues were also treated harshly by the church and the state. Homosexuality continues to be seen as 'abnormal' by some religions and is outlawed in some countries. Gradually, many conditions once managed by religions or the state have been medicalised by assigning diagnoses and treatments, but not always to the benefit of those who were diagnosed. Many harmful medical and surgical treatments were devised to treat various sexual 'disorders' that are now considered normal.

Perhaps the question is: what *should* be diagnosed as a disease? In our efforts to diagnose every deviation from 'normal' so that it can be forced into the disease–illness paradigm, and therefore one day cured, we haven't asked the important question: is this a net good for the person involved? Doctors don't always think this through. They're keen to get the diagnosis part of the paradigm right, but don't always consider the basic philosophical question regarding the purpose of making a diagnosis: will the person be better off?

Medicine is full of examples where this endeavour has failed or is currently in question.

Autism

Autism has long been considered a disease, complete with associated 'impairments' (behaviours), with the aim of finding the cure and eradicating it. Is this a noble pursuit? Not necessarily. It has stigmatised people and led to failed, harmful treatments. Questions have been raised about whether autism is a disorder that must be treated or something that represents a natural variant that should be *accommodated* by society. Is the cost to individual identity and dignity from being labelled as impaired, and therefore something outside of normal, outweighed by the special provisions that accompany the label? And are those special provisions effective in improving quality of life? The harms from labelling a person as autistic can be considerable, not only for the person who must carry the label with them forever, separating them from 'normal' people and being told they are disabled, but also for the parents, whose child has now been changed from 'difficult' to 'disordered'.

Is it possible to receive the supports required for their behaviours without the label?

Has the increase in the numbers of people diagnosed as autistic simply been the result of our desire to diagnose, and an *assumption* that it's beneficial? The difficulty in whether to label someone as autistic has been demonstrated by those whose job it is to decide. The official diagnostic psychiatric bible (the *Diagnostic and Statistical Manual*, commonly known as the *DSM*) only recognised it as a disorder in 1980, and the diagnostic criteria have changed with every edition since.

This isn't to deny that it's possible to diagnose people with a certain pattern of behaviours as autistic, we're just asking whether the harms of the label have been sufficiently considered, and whether the label helps everybody who has it.

Many behavioural and psychological conditions have been diagnosed over the years resulting in no benefit, and sometimes in imprisonment, medical harms and, paradoxically, psychological harms.

Pain

Pain is a common symptom and an important concern for everybody. But attempts to overmedicalise pain, even expected or 'normal' pain, have also resulted in harms. The current opioid epidemic has its origins in treating pain as a disease or an unnatural condition that must be eradicated. While this sounds appealing on the surface, like a lot of things in medicine it's just not that simple, and unintended consequences commonly arise. Doctors thought there was an epidemic of undertreated pain, but they never properly considered the paradoxical harms that would come from overtreating it.

Pain is a normal response to a noxious stimulus, and it has an important role in maintaining health. Beyond the obvious benefit of avoiding potential or real harms, such as putting your hand on a very hot stove, pain has other benefits. After surgery, it heightens our awareness of the surgical wound and the need to protect it. Suppressing pain too much after surgery reduces awareness, and can reduce the drive to breathe so that people can inhale food or vomit, fail to properly inflate or clear their lungs, or simply stop breathing. People die from receiving too much pain relief after surgery. This can occur in otherwise well people who are having elective surgery and are being treated on normal hospital wards. It's a particular problem for people prone to breathing problems from conditions such as sleep apnoea, which stops them breathing for repeated short periods while they're asleep. Suppressing pain to the extent that it reduces the drive to breathe is another way that opioids can cause death. All this is attributable to seeing pain as 'abnormal'.

Low back pain

Most adults will have non-serious low back pain at some point in their lifetime. About one in four people will have back pain at any one time, and many of us will have recurrent episodes. It can almost be considered a normal everyday part of life, and that's exactly how it was viewed throughout history. Most people didn't pay much attention to back pain, let alone consider it a medical condition, and almost no one suffered any disabling permanent problems; it was just a part of life.

Low back pain gets better quickly whether it's treated or not. This has been shown in a study that included every single trial investigating treatments such as medicines or physical treatments for acute low back pain and testing them against placebo, no treatment, usual care or another treatment. The results were astonishing. It didn't matter if the treatment was placebo, nothing, usual care or the specific treatment under study, everyone improved by about the same amount across the same time period, meaning that none of the treatments were any better, on average, than doing nothing.

It's proven very difficult to shift the current thinking away from the disease–illness paradigm to a more constructive way of managing the problem – providing assurance that the pain is not serious, accepting that it's a normal part of life, and promoting resilience and positive health. The disease–illness paradigm forces the doctor into a course of action based on a 'reductionist' approach, where the doctor narrows down all possible causes in the pursuit of a single specific diagnosis or cause. Some serious conditions certainly need to be considered when someone complains of low back pain, but these are rare (less than 1 per cent) and easy to detect or rule out in most cases with a thorough clinical assessment.

Low back pain is so common that many people have it every day but never seek a diagnosis or treatment. More than half *never* seek care. But others are consumed by it, focusing on every minor change in their symptoms, endlessly interpreting its significance. They worry about its implications and what the impact will be on their future. Their lives can virtually come to a standstill because of the pain or, specifically, because of their interpretation of and reaction to the pain.

People with low back pain are often fearful of movement. They fear that moving will make the problem worse or will reinjure their back, and they assume the problem will inevitably get worse. Such beliefs, and other non-physical factors such as depression and low job satisfaction, are highly predictive of becoming disabled from back pain.

Rather than settling for a non-serious or 'non-specific' diagnosis of low back pain, overdiagnosis and overtreatment of low back pain is rife – and it's an industry. Back pain represents a major part of the medical–industrial complex involving drug-makers, pharmacists, radiologists, hospital owners, surgical device-makers, an array of different types of doctors and many other health practitioners, including physiotherapists, chiropractors and psychologists.

Here's how it works. If, like many people, you have low back pain and are concerned by it, you may see a doctor or another healthcare professional. Instead of saying 'I know not', they will recommend a test. Whereas in the past this was likely to be a plain X-ray, these days this is more likely to be a CT scan or MRI scan. Depending on your age, the report may indicate lots of normal age-related changes and will contain lots of medical words that sound worrying but are likely to be irrelevant. Because they sound worrying, this might lead to more tests or a referral to see a specialist.

In any case, the doctor or other health professional will be uncomfortable telling you they don't know what the specific cause is. Instead, they may give you the preferred diagnosis of their particular discipline or specialty. Chiropractors might diagnose your problem as spinal malalignment and physiotherapists as a weakness of your core muscles. Radiologists might diagnose facet joint arthritis, pain specialists might diagnose neuropathic pain, and surgeons might diagnose instability or nerve compression due to degenerative discs.

Not surprisingly, each of these diagnostic labels has a matching treatment that's provided by the branch of health care that provided the diagnosis. Most, if not all, have either been proven in rigorous scientific trials not to make people better, or have not yet been subjected to rigorous trials. The mere labelling reinforces the idea that there's a 'problem' that must be treated.

Despite many published guidelines on back pain that recommend a more hands-off approach, studies have shown that doctors and other health practitioners have difficulty following these guidelines, resulting in too many tests, referrals and treatments rather than saying 'I know not'.

We've discussed the harms of pain medicines, but what's worse is that the evidence for painkillers actually 'killing' pain in the first place is weak. Paracetamol (Panadol, Panamax or acetaminophen) has been shown to be no more effective than placebo for back pain, and studies of opioids have shown little long-term benefit for chronic pain and a consistently high rate of adverse effects. They're also no more effective than simple, non-opioid medicines such as non-steroidal anti-inflammatory drugs (Voltaren, ibuprofen). Pregabalin (Lyrica), a drug that treats 'nerve pain', is commonly used for back pain, particularly when accompanied by pain radiating down the leg, but has been shown to be no more effective than placebo in at least three high-quality trials to date. In addition, there's a substantial risk of side effects particularly among older people. It has also contributed to deaths, particularly when taken together with opioids.

Avoid practitioners with a special interest in low back pain

A groundbreaking study that Rachelle performed in the late 1990s evaluated a mass media campaign in the state of Victoria, Australia. It was designed to change common misconceptions about back pain among the general public, including doctors. The brainchild of the Victorian WorkCover Authority (VWA), its slogan was 'Don't take back pain lying down'. It resulted from the VWA's inability to curb the rising costs of workers' compensation claims for low back pain, which had tripled in the previous decade.

The campaign was mainly delivered via television commercials aired during peak viewing times, such as major state or national sporting events. The campaign messages were simple and clear, and provided evidence-based and unambiguous advice directed towards staying active and exercising, not resting for prolonged periods, and remaining at work. The ads also emphasised that most people didn't need to get their back X-rayed and that there was a lot that people with back pain themselves could do to manage the problem. The messages were delivered by a variety of people from doctors and other health professionals, international experts on low back pain, Australian sporting icons including the cricketer Merv Hughes (a well-known sufferer of back pain), and well-known Australian comedians.

Rachelle's study measured the Victorian general population's beliefs before, during and after the campaign, and compared these with the beliefs of the population in the neighbouring state of New South Wales, where the campaign wasn't aired. It also compared the knowledge, attitudes and beliefs of Victorian doctors, as well as how they would treat people with low back pain before, during and after the campaign, and again compared this with their counterparts in New South Wales. The study found that the campaign was highly effective in shifting both societal and doctors' attitudes towards more evidence-based beliefs about back pain in Victoria, while there was no change at all in the public's or doctors' beliefs in New South Wales. Follow-up studies showed that these changes were sustained as long as five and a half years after the campaign ended.

Beliefs weren't the only thing to change in Victoria. Doctors indicated they would manage back pain using significantly fewer X-rays, and less bed rest and keeping people home from work. There was also a clear decline in the number of workers' compensation claims for low back pain, as well as a significant drop in the duration of time off work for a claim and an overall 20 per cent reduction in the total workers' compensation costs.

Societal beliefs had shifted irrespective of the type of work people did, their income or education, whether they were born in Australia or overseas, their age or gender, whether or not they had a history of back pain and even whether or not they remembered seeing the TV ads. Everyone, it seems, changed their beliefs.

And now for the kicker. One group of people wasn't affected by the campaign at all. Before the campaign, doctors in both states who indicated that they had a special interest in back pain had poorer beliefs about back pain than doctors without a special interest. The Victorian back doctors did not shift their beliefs in the slightest over the course of the campaign. Compared with all other doctors, they were significantly more likely to believe that complete bed rest and avoidance of work is appropriate for people with acute low back pain and that imaging such as X-rays is useful. The bottom line? If you have low back pain, avoid seeing doctors who declare a special interest in it. This is likely to apply to other healthcare professionals as well.

The campaign and its evaluation, which both won many awards including the coveted award for the best paper on low back pain published each year, has now been replicated in one form or another in many other countries, including Scotland, Wales, Canada, Norway and the Netherlands.

Headache

Headache is another common complaint where the patient will often be better off if their doctor says 'I know not'. Like back pain, most headaches have no identifiable cause, and most are transient. Understandably, people with headache want to have their symptoms explained. And doctors feel that it's their role to do that, or at least to rule out sinister causes, which make up only about 0.1 per cent (or 1 in 1000) of all headaches seen in primary care. This can lead the patient down the very similar one-way path of overdiagnosis and overtreatment.

Many findings on neck X-rays, brain scans, blood tests, sinus scans, eye tests and psychiatric screening *could* explain headache. Yet many of the findings on those tests are commonly seen in people without headaches. Instead of considering the unlikely probability that the finding is the *cause* of the headache, doctors often just treat what they see.

Many conditions are overdiagnosed as a result of headache. One interesting current debate is whether headaches can be caused by pineal cysts (the pineal gland lies deep within the centre of the brain and sometimes has benign cysts), and if the cysts should therefore be removed. Some surgeons remove the pineal cyst to treat headaches and some don't. We don't yet know whether surgery is better than doing nothing, because nobody has done the comparative study necessary to answer the question.

We do know that pineal cysts don't grow much over time, and that the larger ones tend to get smaller if left alone. We also know that almost a quarter of people without headaches have a detectable pineal cyst on an MRI scan, and that this rises to 40 per cent in autopsy studies. We also know that nearly everybody will complain of headaches in their lifetime and most people will have at least one headache in any given year. In other words, headaches are common and pineal cysts are common. It's likely that we're assuming causation between two common and frequently overlapping but unrelated events.

The problem of headache and medicalisation has been compounded by the newly diagnosed condition of medication overuse headache, now considered one of the most common causes of headache. This is caused by taking too much headache medication. Basically, our diagnosis and treatment of headache has led to more headaches, and a new diagnosis. Doctors have a treatment for this new condition; it involves stopping the medication but adding some new ones.

Doctors are all scared of missing diagnoses, but they can often rule out important diagnoses very easily by taking a good history and performing a thorough examination, without subjecting every patient to a series of tests. Tests are likely to show up findings that will be treated even if they're not causing a problem. Even if a doctor feels comfortable in having ruled out a serious condition, they may still feel a desire to label it. In fact, everything depends on it: the doctor's reputation (indeed, medicine's reputation as the answer to all our health problems), the patient's wishes, the doctor's income, and the income of everyone in the medical–industrial complex. The label is the patient's ticket into the medical system.

The part about the doctor's reputation is important. It's not just their reputation among their patients and peers, but their sense of value to society, and the justification for their chosen craft and the investments they've made in achieving their position and status. To say 'I know not' to a patient seeking relief *seems* like it goes against medical training. But the health of many patients can be improved, or simply 'less harmed', by a doctor saying 'I know not'. This powerful message can avoid patients going down the one-way road that leads to overtesting, overdiagnosis and their resulting harms.

When the best care might be doing nothing

So far we've covered the harms that result from doctors' unwillingness to say 'I know not' when making a diagnosis. Sometimes, however, the diagnosis is clear – it's not a case of doctors chasing a diagnosis or unnecessarily labelling a person. But when it comes to treatment, doctors are still unwilling to say 'I know not' and to refrain from treating the patient when that might be the best approach. When there's no good treatment or uncertainty regarding the effectiveness of the treatments that are available, no treatment may be best.

Sometimes, even for serious conditions such as life-threatening cancers, there is no good treatment. A cure is deemed impossible but somehow patients still undergo 'heroic' attempts at surgery for tumours that can't be removed, or chemotherapy for cancers in the terminal stages. The problem is that while these approaches *sound* heroic, they may not be logical choices. If the treatment carries risk, which nearly all treatments do, and offers no chance for improvement in life expectancy, symptoms or quality of life, it's not a good choice for the patient. It's also a waste of resources that could be better used elsewhere.

If a treatment, when tested on many people, on average results in no benefit and increased harm, it shouldn't be used. The *probability* (most likely outcome, based on studies of many people) for any individual is that it won't help them. Within the study group, however, some people improved and suffered no harm, while others may have been harmed terribly – not every person shows the same, average result. In such instances, doctors and patients may not objectively balance the probabilities of benefit and harm. Instead, they tend to focus on and inflate the chance of benefit, while ignoring or discounting the chance of harm. The patient would most likely still be better off with no treatment, but they or their doctor don't see it that way. They are buying lottery tickets – they only see the windfall and don't notice the cost.

Another reason doctors recommend ineffective treatments is that it's the path of least resistance, either because it's quicker and simpler or because it aligns with patient expectations or what the doctor *thinks* the patient expects. When prescribing antibiotics for the common cold or flu (both viral infections, against which antibiotics are ineffective), doctors are taking the easy way out. They don't properly consider the risk of a drug reaction, diarrhoea from killing good gut bacteria, and the development of resistant bacteria.

But many of the decisions made by doctors every day are shrouded in uncertainty regarding their relative risks and benefits. Sometimes that uncertainty has been manufactured to promote ongoing treatment. The drug industry, just like the tobacco industry, will sow doubt by using an opinion piece or a low-quality study that opposes current thinking that's unfavourable to their drug. This manufactured doubt implies that there are 'two sides to the story' or that 'the area remains controversial'. When this occurs, rather than basing their decisions on the balance of probabilities, it's easier for doctors to recognise that there's some uncertainty. This gives them enough room to justify treatment. Even the doctors prescribing antibiotics for an obvious viral infection can say 'There's a chance this could be bacterial' and thus treatable with antibiotics.

Ian sees this regularly in his practice as a trauma surgeon treating people with broken bones and torn tendons. There's now good evidence that many injuries, such as Achilles tendon ruptures; common ankle, shoulder and wrist fractures; and even many spinal and pelvic fractures can (and should) be treated without surgery. But every patient is treated as an individual, no two fractures are the same, and there's always *some* degree of uncertainty about the outcome. He often sees patients who have had these injuries treated with surgery and then suffered complications as a direct result of the unnecessary surgery.

The only time Ian's hospital has been sued for his treatment was early in his career, when a patient developed an infection after surgery to repair a torn Achilles tendon. For many years now, he and many other surgeons have been treating these injuries without surgery, because the results are very good and the known complications of surgery (including infection) can be avoided. At the time, though, he didn't know, so he fell into the trap of 'When in doubt, operate'.

* * *

Avoiding unnecessary treatment is not avoiding responsibility. Failure to treat isn't the same as failure to care. Often the reason behind a doctor's bias towards treating versus not treating, is that they don't see *not* treating as an option. When told that their preferred treatments are ineffective, doctors will often respond: 'What else do you expect us to do? We have to do *some*thing'.

They're often blind to the alternative of *not* doing the treatment – they just don't see it as an option. But any decision between treatment options based on the balance of benefit and harm includes the option of not intervening at all. Just like any treatment option, not treating someone also has potential benefits and harms that can be weighed up. And when explained to the patient in those terms, and delivered with compassion and assurance that the situation can be reassessed in the near future, avoiding treatment might be the best thing for the patient. Not treating can be a success, not a failure. It can be good management and avoids unnecessarily exposing patients to harm.

* * *

By saying 'I know not' and providing assurance and explanation *alone*, a doctor can de-medicalise when medicalisation is not in the best interests of the patient. They can uncouple the patient from the medical merry-go-round and return them to their normal life and normal job. This way, patients can rely on their resilience and their social supports to cope with the predicaments that life has dealt them. The doctor may also be saving them some money, some stress and some unnecessary harm.

6

Birth and death

Hippocratic Oath: I will respect the privacy of my patients, for their problems are not disclosed to me that the world may know. Most especially must I tread with care in matters of life and death. If it is given me to save a life, all thanks. But it may also be within my power to take a life; this awesome responsibility must be faced with great humbleness and awareness of my own frailty. Above all, I must not play at God.

'Life is short, and art long'
– Hippocrates

'In Scotland, where I was born, death was seen as imminent. In Canada, where I trained, it was thought inevitable. In California, where I now live, it's seen as optional.'
– Ian Morrison, futurist

Together, birth and death take up a large portion of total healthcare spending. In developed countries, nearly all births take place in a hospital, and nearly everyone gets medical treatment in the weeks and months leading up to death, often in hospital.

'Treading with care in matters of life and death' is where medicine has clearly diverged from the Hippocratic Oath. Just as many of the predicaments of life have been medicalised, so too have these two most natural things in the world. Medicalising birth and death isn't the same as treading with *care* in matters of life and death, not by a long shot. In examining this pledge of the Oath, we will point out where doctors have failed to 'tread with care' in matters of life and death, including the area of euthanasia, and we will discuss the lack of 'humbleness and awareness of our own frailty' in medicine.

The medicalisation of birth

Historically, births were managed exclusively by laywomen and didn't involve doctors. Childbirth was considered a normal life event. Doctors were initially involved in births in the home but by the early 20th century birth had become a mainly hospital-based procedure. Hospitals were still, however, dangerous places for birth, due to a high risk of infection. Even at the time Semmelweis was promoting handwashing to reduce infection, many women preferred to give birth at home because of the high rate of death associated with hospital birth. Advances in sanitation and nutrition over the past 200 years, as well as the advent of antibiotics in the 1930s, led to a decrease in deaths associated with birth and early childhood.

Although many medical advances have been positive for childbirth, such as better methods of pain relief, blood transfusion and the use of caesarean section for complicated pregnancies, some of the interventions used by doctors have been less helpful. Most births in hospitals occur according to guidelines and protocols that doctors have written. While written with the good intention of ensuring a safer delivery for both baby and mother, these 'rules' tend to favour interventions such as inducing or enhancing labour with drugs, breaking the water sac surrounding the foetus (the amniotic membrane), and caesarean sections.

Monitoring for foetal distress

In labour, the foetus can be monitored for 'distress' with a device called an electronic foetal monitor or cardiotocograph (CTG). This provides a live reading of the foetal heartbeat and contractions of the uterus. When used appropriately, electronic foetal monitoring is a useful screening tool for detecting foetal distress and can reduce harms to the foetus. But research has shown that when used unnecessarily, it increases the chance of a caesarean section without reducing the chance of foetal death. Why, when objective scientific studies tell us the opposite, do we tend to intervene? This might be because of uncertainty, but doctors also intervene in these instances because they fear an imperfect outcome and the threat of litigation. The medical paradigm is risk averse and can therefore tend towards finding a 'trigger' or a reason to intervene. Fear of litigation in particular is often cited as a major driver for increased intervention rates in pregnancy and labour, and potentially more caesarean section operations.

Giving oxygen to premature babies

Another procedure that until recently was widespread is giving oxygen to newborn babies with low oxygen levels, a common problem with premature birth. In theory, it sounds good to help babies with breathing problems, but studies comparing newborns given oxygen with those given normal room air showed that the babies given oxygen were more likely to develop problems such as blindness and were more likely to die. Oxygen is now only given in certain more severe cases, and the dosage of oxygen supplied is closely controlled because too much can be harmful. This is a clear example of a medical intervention being introduced based on good intentions alone. It was *assumed* that it would help without any evidence to support its use, and it led to unintended and harmful consequences.

To cut or not to cut

The birth process itself has been medicalised the most. The use of an episiotomy, an incision in the perineum to cut open the birth canal at the opening of the vagina, was routinely used from around the mid-20th century to prevent the spontaneous tears that can occur during childbirth. Sometimes these tears can be severe, requiring surgical repair and time to heal.

It *sounds* like a good idea if the baby's progress through the birth canal is blocked. It seems logical that cutting open the birth canal should facilitate birth as well as prevent a spontaneous tear. But determining whether the baby's head will fit through without an episiotomy is very subjective. And when things are subjective or uncertain, doctors tend to act, which is why episiotomies were commonly performed in many hospitals. In the United States during the 1970s, for example, they were used in nearly two-thirds of all vaginal births.

While it remains debatable, of course, there's some evidence that natural tears may hurt less, bleed less and heal quicker than an episiotomy, which means that when episiotomies were commonly used they may have been providing little or no benefit and a lot of harm, including pain and scarring of the vagina. While some claim that episiotomies might reduce late complications of childbirth such as vaginal prolapse and urinary incontinence, the available evidence does not support this.

Current Australian guidelines recommend against the routine use of episiotomy except in certain situations, such as to hasten delivery of a distressed foetus, but the use of episiotomies continues to vary widely between doctors, hospitals and countries. In one Australian state, the hospital with the highest rate performs 20 times more episiotomies than the one with the lowest rate. It's also more common in private hospitals, where medical intervention rates remain high overall.

Forceps

Forceps are curved metal clamps inserted through the vagina to clamp (sorry, 'cradle') the baby's head during birth and bring the baby out. At one stage, the use of forceps and episiotomy was promoted to eliminate the 'pushing' stage of childbirth. Its use also rose with the increased use of epidurals, which hamper the mother's ability to push.

Forceps can cause harm to both the baby and the mother and they were overused. The misuse and overuse of forceps during delivery has led them being banned completely in some hospitals. Although forceps can still play a role in some situations, their use has significantly declined, partly because caesareans are considered safer for difficult deliveries (but also partly due to a lack of obstetricians suitably trained in their use).

Caesarean sections

The WHO has variously put the 'ideal' rate of caesarean section at 10 and 15 per cent. It notes that when caesarean section rates rise towards 10 per cent across a population, the number of maternal and newborn deaths decreases. When they rise above 10 per cent, however, there's no evidence that the mortality rates improve.

In developed countries, however, the rate of caesarean use is rising from an already high level. In Australia and the United States, about 33 per cent of babies are born via caesarean section. Worldwide the average is about 30 per cent. The rate varies a lot geographically, both within and between countries. In China and Brazil, the rate is about 50 per cent, while in some developing countries, such as Ethiopia, Chad, South Sudan and Niger, the rates are less than 2 per cent, signifying underuse. In some countries there are huge discrepancies between caesarean sections by economic status. In Peru, for example, more than half the pregnant women in the richest fifth of the population have caesarean sections, while the rate falls to well below 10 per cent for the poorest fifth.

The rise in caesarean rates has been justified for many reasons, such as increasing obesity rates and rising maternal age, but most of them don't stack up. Even the more traditional reasons, like breech presentation (when the foetus presents with the buttocks or feet first rather than the head first), failure for labour to progress and previous caesarean section, aren't necessarily correct. Breech-presentation births can be safely trialled with vaginal delivery first. 'Failure to progress' is overdiagnosed. The popular dictum 'once a caesarean always a caesarean', coined in the 1970s when the rate of caesarean section tripled, has long been challenged in the absence of such compelling reasons as a high risk of bleeding. They are still commonly recommended, however, most likely due to a rise in litigation rates.

Another important reason for the rise in caesarean section is maternal request. A 2021 review of 5 million total births across 14 countries found that the rate of maternally requested caesareans ranged between 0.2 and 42 per cent, with large variations across studies. The majority of this variation was explained by the differing economic status of the country, but not in the way that you might expect. The overall number of maternally requested caesareans was 11 times higher in upper-middle-income countries than in high-income countries. The authors postulated that the stronger healthcare systems in high-income countries might mean that caesareans are less likely in the absence of valid indications other than a woman's preference.

Why worry if caesareans are overused? Surely they are safe, and if there's any doubt at all, shouldn't we do a caesarean section just in case? As usual, the harms are often not sufficiently considered. Although caesareans are a lot safer than they used to be, they are by no means risk-free. A caesarean is still an operation, and all the usual risks that accompany any operation – including anaesthetic complications, wound infections, wound breakdown and blood clots – still apply. More specific complications include possible excessive bleeding, infection of the uterus, urinary infection, and damage to surrounding structures such as the ureter (which connects the kidney to the bladder) and bladder. In rare instances, complications can lead to the need to remove the uterus (hysterectomy), a devastating outcome if the woman is planning on future pregnancies. In Australia between 2003 and 2014, six out of 10 000 women giving birth had a caesarean and hysterectomy during the same hospital admission.

It's the complications that occur later, however, that are often discounted. After mum and baby have gone home and no longer need to see the doctor, problems can and do occur. Firstly, the uterine scarring that results from caesareans can lead to serious complications in five to seven out of 1000 later births due to uterine rupture. This is why the main reason for having a caesarean is having had one previously – a snowball effect. Both placenta praevia (a low-lying placenta) and placenta accreta (where the placenta grows into the uterus and doesn't peel away) can result in bleeding, and the latter often requires surgery. These scarring issues make each subsequent caesarean section surgery more difficult, and thus more prone to complications. There can also be persistent pain at the site of surgery, incisional endometriosis (growth of the lining of the uterus, the endometrium, in the caesarean scar), thickening of the wall of the uterus, bowel obstructions due to surgical scarring and numbness around the scar.

In addition to the complications that can arise for the mother, adverse effects have also been reported in the baby. These include depressed immune function, obesity, respiratory compromise, poor maternal–infant bonding and breastfeeding difficulties. There's also a cost factor: caesarean sections are more expensive than vaginal births.

Bringing on or enhancing labour

Most births in Australia now involve medical intervention of some kind. Apart from the one-third that are caesarean births, around half of labours are induced or enhanced in some way. For example, doctors think that the cervix, which widens to allow delivery, should dilate by 1 centimetre per hour. If it doesn't, they use that rule (another example of medicalising) to justify intervening, but it turns out that it's fine if the cervix takes a little longer to dilate.

Induction of labour is also overdone. In Australia between 2004 and 2018, around 43 per cent of first-time mothers aged 20–34 whose baby's gestational age at birth was between 37 and 41 weeks had their labour induced. Although inductions are probably only beneficial for pregnancies well past their due date, they're commonly used for any delivery, and it has been estimated that most of them are unnecessary. Can they cause harm? Yes, but probably the most important harm is that induction often leads to a caesarean section, another example of how one intervention leads to another.

Medical interventions in the birth process have played a role in improving survival and health outcomes for mothers and babies, but individually, some of these interventions may cause harm without benefit. Broader research has also shown that overall, births with interventions have a higher rate of complications for both the mother and the baby, even allowing for the fact that some of the mothers who had interventions were sicker.

The WHO has made recommendations that aim to make childbirth a more positive experience by transferring the power and control over birth to the mother and creating a culture of respect for her. It specifically indicates problems with the medicalisation of birth, including the use of language that pushes women into accepting more interventions (e.g. terms like 'failure to progress', which is commonly used to justify interventions) and the overuse of certain interventions. It recommends changing the birth model away from one framed in terms of 'risk' towards a more positive one centred on the birthing woman and her informed choices.

The medicalisation of dying

Not so long ago, most people died at home, in familiar surroundings, comfortably and surrounded by loved ones. When asked, people still say they would rather die at home. Today, only about a quarter of all deaths occur at home while another quarter occur in hospices, nursing homes and other institutions. The remaining half occur in hospitals, and people who die in hospitals often undergo painful treatments in the doctors' futile attempts to avoid the inevitable.

In intensive care in particular, the focus of the doctors has been less on human suffering and dignity and more on the struggle to maintain vital signs. Around 20 per cent of all deaths occur in intensive care units, which is one reason the financial cost of death is so high. Intensive care costs in the last month of life make up around 80 per cent of the total costs incurred in the final year of life. Around 30 per cent of the US Medicare budget is spent on the 5 per cent of recipients who die each year.

One of the problems is that there is uncertainty among doctors regarding the role of some treatments, which often leads to a 'give it a go' mentality. The lack of guidelines or protocols for treating dying or very sick patients doesn't help. The problem is made even worse in situations where the dying person is unconscious or unable to discuss treatment options due to dementia. The tendency in those cases is to try anything to 'save' or extend life, with little regard to quality of life.

We need to divert the focus from avoiding death to ensuring a 'good death'. A good death means one that's accepted and comfortable, with conflicts resolved and according to personal preferences – for example, surrounded by loved ones at home.

Everybody dies – it's the only inescapable part of life. The

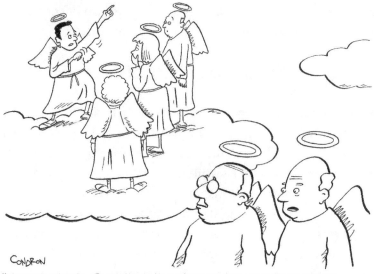

"NOBODY WANTS TO HEAR OUR STORIES ABOUT DEATH FROM NATURAL CAUSES."

problem with medicalising death is that attributing any death to disease or injury implies that it could possibly have been prevented by medical treatments. This makes death look like failure for doctors. The inevitability of death isn't always factored into the medical model of care. The other thing not often factored in is the patient's wishes. Doctors and nurses say they give dying patients much more aggressive treatments than they would want for themselves in the same situation. Terminally ill doctors spend less time getting treatments and less time in hospital than the people they once treated.

The idea behind aggressive treatments for patients with incurable cancer is that the period of time spent having chemotherapy (often associated with a temporarily poor *quality* of life) is worth it if it extends life (increased *quantity* of life). It's obviously a difficult decision, but the premise may not always be true.

Doctors owe it to their patients to discuss their preferences, because it turns out better for them and better for society. One study showed that simply having end-of-life discussions improved the quality of death for the patients with cancer, and significantly lowered use of heroic intensive care treatments, thereby also saving a lot of money.

Unless patients are properly informed and asked, they will tend to hand over responsibility for managing their own death and dying to the doctors, who don't always know what to do with it. Doctors end up approaching it like any other disease they treat: an enemy that is to be feared, defeated and controlled, not respected and accepted. For a doctor, allowing death to occur is to fail at caring. But death and dying are part of life, not the opposite of life, and a good death is part of a good life.

Society's role in the medicalisation of dying

With the withdrawal of the influence of community and religion, modern culture and science itself – with their emphasis on individualism, secularism and disease – may have played a part in the medicalisation of dying. This has taken away the meaning and the means of comfort from death and contributed to a fear of death. We have also allowed a culture of defiance and denial of death to rise, seeing death as something to battle and therefore dying as a sign of individual weakness and defeat.

Culture may have changed, but it's doctors who have taken up responsibility for death and applied it to their disease-based care models by treating death as a disease process, further increasing the fear of death.

The specialty of palliative care was started in response to the problems of medicalising dying, but the doctors were put in charge of this too, so palliative care itself has been medicalised, and non-medical ways of managing death have been devalued. As with birth, doctors struggle to balance technical intervention and a humanistic approach to their dying patients.

The role of social factors in dealing with death is managed within a medical framework. The focus is on symptom management as a surrogate for quality of death, on pain as a surrogate for all suffering, and therefore on drugs and how best to deliver them (slow release, patches, small infusers, and so on) and on *controlling* the dying process, preferably in a hospital or a hospice rather than at home. Yet the most pressing concerns of dying patients are social and psychological, not symptom management.

US writer and scholar David B Morris summed it up best in his 1998 book *Illness and Culture in the Postmodern Age*: 'dying patients are trapped between two evils: a runaway medical technology of ventilators, surgeries and organ transplants that can keep bodies alive indefinitely and – as if this prospect were not frightening enough – an understandable but reckless public clamour for physician-assisted suicide as the only alternative to such ignominious physician-assisted suffering'.

The false debate about 'physician-assisted' dying

There's definitely a debate to be had about the preference for death over severe suffering. But while some may see the death of a patient at the hand of a physician as the very epitome of medicine's control over life, that doesn't mean it's bad. We use the term medicalisation negatively throughout this book, but there are many instances where medicine has taken over control of processes to the benefit of society and the individuals within it.

The point about physician-assisted dying lies in the name – physician-assisted. It refers to a situation where physicians can be seen as facilitators of a *person's* decision to end their own life. That decision is the ultimate in patient autonomy, allowing someone to choose not only to terminate their life, but to have a say in when, where and how it occurs.

The real debate is whether people should be able to make these decisions, rather than whether physicians should help patients die. Knowing that physicians are on hand to make it easier will of course influence a person's decision, but it's still the decision itself that's most important. Once a society has deemed it reasonable for a patient to make this decision, there are benefits to having doctors involved, mainly for their technical knowledge. If we have any caution, it would concern the extreme care required in discussing the issue with the patient and what information is taken into account when they make their decision.

It isn't helpful to label physician-assisted death as 'playing God' – that's an easy way to dismiss it without due consideration. Doctors 'play God' all the time; the question is whether it's beneficial for them to do so.

The doctor's pedestal: our rightful place?

One aspect of 'playing God' deserves much more discussion. Doctors are rarely accused of being humble, with good reason. Doctors are held in very high regard, particularly by their patients, so their control over the decision-making process is tight – in some cases, total. This opens the door for corruption of that power, particularly when doctors start believing they deserve adulation and start to lose their humility.

Interestingly, but perhaps not surprisingly, male doctors have often been shown to be more confident in their abilities, despite often being less competent than female doctors at the same tasks. Rachelle first became aware of this dichotomy in one of her earliest studies, which invited about 800 primary care physicians in Ontario, Canada, to complete a mailed questionnaire asking them how they would manage five hypothetical patients with musculoskeletal complaints as well as their confidence in managing them. Ironically, the research team was led by a male doctor and the rest of the team were women. The study found that for almost every aspect of care (e.g. prescribing medications, giving injections), the male doctors were more confident in providing that care. But when assessing the appropriateness of the care, more female doctors selected the recommended management options.

The 'hero' surgeon

Surgeons, by the nature of their job, are prone to being arrogant. They make irreversible decisions and have to live with them, so it's easier to reassure patients (as well as themselves) by being certain that theirs were the right decisions, whatever the outcome.

Some surgeons are considered heroes because they do operations no one else is doing, but the reason no one else is doing them is often because there's evidence that the operation is futile and won't benefit the patient. These operations are often bigger and more difficult than other operations, like attempting to remove a brain tumour deemed inoperable, but that doesn't mean they're helpful. To justify the lack of competition from colleagues, the surgeon can see themselves as the hero – the only one brave and skilled enough to do this procedure, *particularly* in the face of the terrible odds for success. This also allows the 'hero' surgeon to justify a very high fee.

It's easy to see how a desperate patient could fall for this story and submit to the procedure. It's an appealing narrative to go for the long shot – in a movie, it would work nearly every time, but in real life it usually ends up making things worse. A lack of regulation regarding the evidence required for surgical procedures doesn't help, but neither does a lack of humility in the surgeon.

The 'overcaring' oncologist

Sometimes doctors use their control of the treatment decision to *under*treat, which also results in harm. It's known, for example, that some oncologists use subtherapeutic (ineffective) doses of chemotherapy to save the patient from experiencing side effects. Despite these good intentions, this may also mean that they're not curing people who could be cured. There's no logic in reducing harms if the benefit is lost in the process.

In 2016, a NSW government enquiry into off-label prescribing of chemotherapy was initiated because a senior oncologist had been administering non-standard chemotherapy (i.e. non-recommended drugs and/or lower doses than recommended by established guidelines) when treating patients with head and neck and colorectal cancer with the intention of curing them. According to the expert panel that advised the enquiry, 'very simply and consistently … this was off-protocol. This was so divorced, from the evidence … This was off the radar'. The oncologist believed that his approach could improve the tolerability and reduce the side effects of the treatment, but the enquiry found no evidence to support this contention.

* * *

Doctors have accepted the pedestal they have been placed on as their rightful place – they often feel no need to justify it because everybody already believes it. Medicine is a field full of probabilities and uncertainty, where doctors are expected and willing to provide certainty. These two situations don't mix well; humility is the ingredient that allows them to mix.

There's evidence that the proportion of people dying in hospital is declining, and that the proportion dying in a hospice or at home is increasing. There's also evidence that the proportion of women choosing to deliver their babies at home is increasing and, after decades of rising, the rates of caesarean section use in the United States, the bellwether for overtreatment, has plateaued over recent years and is falling in many states.

7

Treating the problem

Hippocratic Oath: I will remember that I do not treat a fever chart, a cancerous growth, but a sick human being, whose illness may affect the person's family and economic stability. My responsibility includes these related problems, if I am to care adequately for the sick.

'The map is not the territory'
– Alfred Korzybski, Polish–US philosopher

In orthopaedics, we often say 'Treat the patient, not the X-ray'. The most *important* outcome is the one that's most important to the patient and reflects the goals of treatment. These include not dying, good quality of life, and relief of pain or improvement in performing daily activities. In contrast to this are *surrogate* outcomes, which are peripheral or secondary to, and often used instead of, the most important outcomes. A *surrogate* outcome in someone with diabetes might be, for example, their blood sugar level, while the *important* outcome might be preventing the complications of diabetes, such as blindness or kidney failure.

The surrogate outcome and its poster child flecainide

A well-known example of treating the surrogate outcome instead of the most important outcome was the use of flecainide following a heart attack. In the period after a heart attack, the sufferer can die suddenly of an abnormal heart rhythm called an arrhythmia. To prevent these sudden deaths, doctors would give drugs that reduce arrhythmia (called anti-arrhythmics) such as flecainide. Superficially, this makes sense, but we hope by now that you're thinking about the possible unintended consequences that reducing arrhythmias has for deaths (the *important* outcome), rather than its effects on heart rhythm (the *surrogate* outcome).

The effectiveness of flecainide was proven in randomised trials that gave some participants the drug and some participants placebo pills. All the participants were hooked up to continuous heart monitors, and those who took the flecainide clearly had fewer arrhythmias. Death wasn't an outcome in these original studies, but it easily could have been.

Based on these trials, the drug was approved by the FDA and was used across the United States on hundreds of thousands of heart attack patients in the 1980s. Although an association with lower mortality (fewer deaths) had not been established, doctors felt that a randomised trial to test this would be unethical, given the drugs clearly worked, even if only on the surrogate outcome.

Fortunately, some researchers who weren't convinced about the value of flecainide later did similar studies, but with the death rate as the main outcome. They showed that people were much more likely to die if given flecainide. The rate of death with flecainide was so high, in fact, that they had to stop the trial early to avoid more deaths. Overall, the introduction of these antiarrhythmic drugs was responsible for tens of thousands of deaths in the United States alone, and one estimate is more than 120 000.

Why do researchers use surrogate outcomes? Often it's well intentioned: they believe them to be valid measures of the real outcome of interest, and they're often easier, quicker and/or cheaper to collect. But death isn't that hard to measure, and it's hard to fake. It really should be used as the main endpoint for studies on treatments that are meant to keep you alive. This principle is also important in routine care, where doctors also tend to treat surrogate outcomes.

Treating the numbers not the patient

Doctors tend to like numbers because they're measurable values. If a number lies outside 'normal' they want to bring it into line. This has been termed the 'normalisation heuristic'. A heuristic is a rule of thumb, an approach to problem solving, and normalisation means treating measurable abnormalities to 'correct' or bring them back to what's considered normal.

The normalisation heuristic term was coined by an intensive care specialist, Scott K Aberegg. Intensive care units have provided us with some of the best examples of treating the numbers, not the patient. It was once thought, for example, that tight control of the blood sugar level in critically ill patients in intensive care was important to keep them alive. It sounded like a good idea and it was supported by the collective personal experience of many doctors. It was common practice until a large, randomised trial was published in 2009 that compared tight control of the blood sugars to a more relaxed approach. The study showed that the patients whose blood sugars were controlled were more likely to die: the exact opposite of what everybody thought.

Sometimes, treating the numbers and not the patient refers to treating 'risk factors' for a disease. Risk factors, by themselves, may not be important. Having a risk factor means that someone is *more likely* to develop disease in the future compared to someone without that risk factor, all other things being equal. Some risk factors aren't easily modifiable or treatable, meaning that whatever we do, the risk factor doesn't change. For example, if a woman's mother had breast cancer, then her chance of developing breast cancer is twice that of someone whose mother didn't have breast cancer. Our interest lies in the risk factors that *can* be changed by medical care.

Many risk factors are derived from tests and described in numbers, like a blood test to measure cholesterol, or a bone density test to measure how porous the bones are. While a high cholesterol level or high blood pressure are risk factors for heart attacks and strokes, it should not be assumed that treating these risk factors will fully prevent the heart attack or stroke, or that the treatment won't cause other problems.

Treating the numbers rather than the patient gives us two difficulties. First is the danger of using a surrogate rather than the more important outcomes to determine the effectiveness of treatments. In routine care, it's like a surgeon saying they fixed the fracture although the patient died, or the operation was a success but the patient's symptoms didn't improve. In trials, one problem is that when it will take a long time before the important outcomes can be known, the researchers can instead choose surrogate outcomes that they can measure more quickly. They presume that there will be a tight relationship between the surrogate outcomes and the more important final outcomes, but this is commonly not the case. The second difficulty arises when doctors treat risk factors in the absence of disease.

As we've seen, the definition of 'normal' for many tests is arbitrary, often based on a chosen statistical limit or on the opinion of a committee. Even then, normal ranges vary considerably between individuals, and being outside of an average 'population' normal range may still be normal for some people. The same person can also have widely varying numbers on repeated tests. For example, their blood pressure may vary depending on whether the reading was taken at home or in a doctor's office. Many physiological measures, such as blood pressure, can also vary depending upon the time of day, intake of food and drink, exercise and stress. Even repeating someone's blood pressure in the same environment five minutes later can give a different result. The same applies to blood tests, which can vary with different readers and different laboratories, or with errors in the machines used to measure the test.

Surrogate outcomes in cancer

The use of surrogate outcomes in testing cancer drugs has received a lot of attention over the years, thanks to researchers such as Dr Vinay Prasad, a US haematologist–oncologist. He has examined the use of surrogate outcomes in the approval process for cancer drugs through regulatory bodies such as the FDA.

Cancer drugs are supposed to extend life and/or improve the quality of life. But when they are tested against other drugs, or against placebo, the outcomes used to determine their effectiveness are often surrogates, such as tumour shrinkage, dying from the disease or the disease recurring. On the face of it, these outcomes sound appropriate, but the surrogates used in cancer research are often not tested to see if they correlate with what we *really* want which is better *overall* survival and better quality of life. In fact, surrogate outcomes are often found *not* to correlate with these important outcomes at all.

How can that be? Partly because things like tumour shrinkage or time to progression of cancer don't tell you what's happening to all the tumours in the body, only the ones that are being measured. It also doesn't tell you what happens after it shrinks (does it come back even stronger?) or what other effects the treatment is having on the rest of the body. In a review of surrogate outcomes in cancer research, it was shown that only 16 percent of them were highlight correlated with overall survival.

One study of FDA approvals showed that all drugs given 'accelerated' approval were done so based on surrogate outcomes. This may be reasonable, because the idea of accelerated approval is to get the drugs out there if they show promise, and then continue to collect the data on their real effectiveness later. The problem is that most of the surrogate outcomes used for accelerated approvals were never tested to ensure they were closely correlated with measures of the real outcome, such as overall survival. And when they were tested, they mostly failed. There are even cases of drugs having to be withdrawn after rapid approval because they were later found to be harming people and improving neither survival nor quality of life.

As we saw in chapter 3, PSA testing for prostate cancer raises similar red flags. It's understandable that some patients with prostate cancer picked up by a raised PSA opt for surgery, but they shouldn't have had the test in the first place if it wasn't going to increase their chances of a better outcome. The benefits of removing the prostate, or prostatectomy, are usually measured by lower disease-specific mortality, or its counterpart, higher disease-specific survival. But in people with prostate cancer we should be focused not on saving lives from prostate cancer, but on saving lives full stop.

Correcting anaemia in kidney disease

Chronic kidney disease is a common condition, and most patients who have it also have anaemia (low red blood cell counts) severe enough that it causes weakness, fatigue and shortness of breath. In chronic kidney disease, anaemia occurs due to a deficiency in a hormone produced in the kidneys called erythropoietin (EPO), which regulates the production of red blood cells. Scientists produced EPO in a laboratory, and tests showed that giving it to people with kidney disease increased their red blood cell count. The drug is still commonly used, but the benefits need to be carefully weighed against the potential risks. The treatment works very well at increasing the red blood cell count, but studies of this treatment showed no benefit in quality of life. It also makes the blood thicker, and this resulted in more strokes, heart attacks, blood clots and deaths.

Bypassing or unblocking narrowed arteries

Unblocking or bypassing narrowed arteries is a classic example of treating the surrogate, not the patient. Narrowing of the artery to the brain, the carotid artery, can cause a loss of blood supply to the brain, resulting in a stroke. A procedure to 'bypass' the narrowed artery was developed in the 1970s and used widely for some time in people who had suffered a stroke or who were at risk of stroke because of a narrowed carotid artery.

The early studies showed good results based on several surrogate outcomes, such as blood flow in the artery and electrical activity in the brain measured by electroencephalogram (EEG). It wasn't until many years later that a high-quality randomised trial compared bypass surgery to leaving the narrowed blood vessel alone. The study found that the surgery didn't improve either of the important outcomes – death and stroke. In fact, some groups fared worse with surgery, and overall the group treated with surgery tended to die earlier. In their keenness to help, doctors relied on evidence using surrogate measures, subjecting many patients to a treatment that may have harmed them and provided no real benefit. These findings are similar to those we saw in chapter 3 with stenting of the coronary artery in people with stable angina.

Stenting is also used to treat narrowing of the main artery to the kidney, a condition called renal artery stenosis. The association between this condition, which results in very high blood pressure, and severe heart disease led to a strong movement in the 1990s to stent this artery. The procedure became very popular based on reported excellent results from studies without a comparison (non-stented) group. Of course, the *association* with cardiac disease immediately makes us think that the narrowing of the renal artery is *causing* the heart disease, but the most likely explanation is simply that the condition that caused the narrowing of the renal artery (atherosclerosis) is the same condition that caused narrowing of the coronary arteries. Several large-scale randomised trials conducted over the past 20 years have shown that people with stented renal arteries did no better than people who were just given the usual drugs. On top of that, the people undergoing the stenting sometimes died of catastrophic complications of the procedure.

The 'subgroup' fallacy

Doctors still think renal artery stenting probably works for some people, because even though there was no benefit from the stenting *on average*, some people stayed the same, some got better and some got worse. Despite this being the case with just about any condition, the interpretation is that there must be a 'subgroup' of people who get better *because of* the stenting.

This way of thinking is a common reaction to studies that show no overall benefit from a treatment: doctors think they can pick the patients who *will* benefit. But this subgroup has not been found in any high-quality trial. Such a subgroup may exist, but we will remain unconvinced unless it's proven in a fair trial.

There are many other examples of flawed thinking when it comes to subgroups. For example, some doctors think they can pick the people who will benefit from vertebroplasty (see chapter 2), even though the trials found no overall benefit from the treatment. Recently, vertebroplasty was approved for re-listing on the government subsidy list in Australia but only for people with a fracture in a specific part of the spine and only if the symptoms have been present for less than three weeks. This decision was based upon what is called 'post-hoc' analyses from a single study – basically fishing trips to look for subgroups that might improve, even though these groups weren't defined before the trial started. This subgroup of people didn't appear to fare any better than the rest of the study population in at least two other randomised placebo-controlled trials. It's also important to note that if there is no net benefit overall and one subgroup really does benefit, then there must be another equally sized subgroup who are made worse, a situation not reflected in the available data.

Beta-blockers

Beta-blocker drugs have been around for a long time and were originally seen as useful for many purposes. They were, however, often used in circumstances where they were later shown to be harmful or ineffective. For example, they were once used in patients undergoing surgical procedures to prevent them from having heart attacks around the time of surgery. In a study that tested this, the beta-blockers were shown to reduce the chance of heart attacks, as expected, but, more importantly, they also increased the overall risk of dying.

More commonly, the reason for prescribing beta-blockers was as first-line drugs for treating high blood pressure. Millions of prescriptions have been written over many decades. The drugs were used because large-scale studies had concluded (correctly) that they lowered blood pressure. There's even evidence that they lowered the rate of some cardiovascular events, such as stroke. It should be noted that blood pressure can't be felt; it's treated in order to make people live longer by avoiding things like heart attacks and strokes. But a 2017 Cochrane review examining all randomised trials of beta-blockers for high blood pressure found that the chance of dying was exactly the same in patients taking a placebo pill. The surrogate outcome (lower blood pressure) was the aim of the treatment and the measure of success, but the important outcome (death) wasn't affected.

Treating thin bones

Another surrogate outcome is thin bones or osteoporosis, which is determined by doing a bone mineral density (BMD) test. This test measures how porous or dense the bones are. Thinning bones are a part of the ageing process. In Australia, based on expert consensus (in the absence of a strong body of evidence), BMD testing is recommended for all people aged 70 and over, but many women in particular are screened earlier, often at the time of menopause. In the United States, the recommendation applies to women aged 65 and older and men 70 and older. Osteoporosis is defined as a bone density that's 2.5 or more units (standard deviations) below the average for a young woman. This cut-off is used by healthcare funders to define osteoporosis and therefore subsidise treatment.

While the risk of fracture approximately doubles for each unit below this cut-off, having a low BMD is not as strongly correlated with having a fracture as some other factors. The strongest factors are increasing age, a previous fracture that occurred after minimum trauma, or a tendency to fall over. Many people with low bone density never fracture, while many people with normal bone density have fractures. Concentrating on BMD as the problem (and therefore only addressing the thin bones) can overshadow real issues, such as reducing falls or preventing people from falling over in the first place. The latter can be done through such simple measures as rearranging rugs, cords and furniture, improving lighting, fixing cataracts and glasses, adjusting medications, and doing exercises to improve balance and muscle and bone strength. The focus on treating the measurable number has meant that the treatment of osteoporosis is sometimes focused solely on expensive and sometimes harmful drugs that act to increase bone density (see chapter 9).

MRI scans

Another seemingly harmless example of treating the numbers and not the patient is the reporting on imaging scans, like MRIs. The problem is that the scans are reported by radiologists, whose skills are defined by how well they pick up deviations from 'normal', without necessarily providing context (e.g. 'normal' age-related changes). This is because of an overemphasis on the consequences of a missed diagnosis, unbalanced by the unintended consequences of overdiagnosis. This system produces very long and detailed reports of scans that may be completely normal.

Because MRI scans are so sensitive, and getting even more sensitive over time, they can detect smaller and smaller changes. Back scans can show thinned, dehydrated and bulging discs, narrowing of the joints that connect each vertebral body to the next, bone spurs, thickening of the bone and ligaments, slight pressure on nerve roots, calcifications, cysts and malalignments. These changes are all normal, and we expect them to be more common as people get older. They're usually not associated with the presence or absence of pain. The radiologist will report all the abnormalities they find, often without accompanying information about the relevance of the findings, including the fact that many are normal for the patient's age. This list of findings contains many scary things for the patient and many things the doctor can be tempted to treat.

The consequence of MRI scanning of backs is that we now have an explosion of invasive treatments in the spine, such as injections of steroids and other substances (blood, for example) into various parts of the spine, radiofrequency treatments, electrical stimulators and surgical procedures, all of which are associated with specific MRI findings. The catch, however, is that these treatments have either been proven not to work (the majority) or remain unproven. They are also costly and can cause harm. The temptation to treat the findings of these scans results from a dangerous combination of scientific misunderstanding, financial incentives and good intentions. It has led doctors to waste resources and harm people, precisely because they didn't remember the Hippocratic pledge – to treat the patient and not the test result.

Follow the money

In 2018, a seemingly uncontentious motion was put before the United Nations – to recommend breastfeeding over milk formula for its health benefits. The problem the motion was trying to address was that many women in developing countries were relying on infant formula rather than breastfeeding, partly because of the advertising from the manufacturers of the infant formulas. This was not only a costly practice, but it removed the positive health and emotional effects of breastfeeding.

Surprisingly, the United States wanted the recommendation softened, which benefited the infant formula industry, but many countries disagreed. One country, Ecuador, was prepared to vote against the amendments suggested by the United States, based on the global health and cost implications. They were immediately threatened with withdrawal of US military aid and with sanctions. Ecuador quickly acquiesced. One should never underestimate the power of big business.

This is a clear example of treating the *dollars*, not the patient. The health industry is the most powerful lobby group in the United States. It includes device and drug companies, insurance companies, hospitals, and imaging companies that are among the largest in the world. The US government has a long history of pro-pharma decisions.

Drug companies have funded grassroots consumer campaigns for their drugs, withheld research that isn't favourable to their drugs, misled doctors and the public about the benefits and harms of their drugs, ghostwritten their own research, and spent billions on marketing and advertising, all to increase sales. The role of the corporation is to maximise profit, not health, and these are just some of the methods they use to achieve that goal.

While it might be easier, and less discomforting, to blame the drug company if drug sales remain inappropriately high after drugs have been proven ineffective or harmful, we should remember that every sale of a prescription drug requires a doctor's signature. Doctors are therefore the ones who are ultimately responsible for the sales figures. They're also responsible for the associated harms, and it's their responsibility to know the risks and benefits when they sign a prescription.

Industry's cosy relationship with doctors

Doctors and the medical industry have always worked closely together, sometimes producing advances that have resulted in large health benefits. But there's another side to the relationship between doctors and the medical industry. Doctors can be offered speaker fees, writing fees, adviser fees, sponsorship of medical education, free samples, indirect kickbacks, conditional research funding, departmental funding (for fellowship training, education, and so on) and direct kickbacks, cash payments and bribes. All the doctor has to do in return is endorse or use the product. Although many medical companies have been found guilty of such practices (including bribery and kickbacks), doctors have rarely been fined for taking such inducements.

This kind of practice isn't confined to the past, but it has changed its form over time. Doctors get paid tens of thousands of dollars for patients they recruit into studies that companies conduct. Doctors and departments still get paid directly for advisory fees, research support and anything that can be construed as education. Large direct and indirect (undeclared payments from patients and industry) incentives to operate or prescribe are a particular problem in developing countries.

Medical representation on guideline committees is also a problem. Many members of these committees have financial ties to industry, often to the producer of the drug or device they are deciding on. Governments and professional societies recognise this as a problem but claim it's impossible to get any or enough experts who don't have financial ties to industry. They also claim that the doctors with the closest ties to industry are also the ones with the most knowledge.

In Australia, the National Health and Medical Research Council won't endorse guidelines that fall outside of its policies with respect to conflicts of interest for committee members. The committees that decide which drugs, devices and tests are recommended or approved for subsidisation by the Australian government also have strict conflict-of-interest policies. Unfortunately, despite quite rigorous rules concerning the introduction of new treatments, there are still many longstanding treatments that were 'grandfathered in' before these rules were set in place and so have never undergone rigorous review. The system can also be corrupted when vested interests push an agenda by appealing directly to the government to overturn or reconsider decisions.

Does money from industry impact clinical practice? We should let the businesses themselves answer. Given that they've been pouring money into these types of activities for a long time, it must be working – they wouldn't be doing it if it weren't profitable. Industry sponsorship adds up to tens of thousands of dollars per year, on average, to physicians in the United States, and although doctors vehemently deny that such amounts could influence their practice, the evidence is that it *does* influence prescribing practices. In Australia, over a six-month period to April 2019, pharmaceutical companies paid a total of $7.3 million to 2775 doctors. Recently, increasing numbers of specialist nurses have received funding, for example to attend international conferences.

While most doctors (and nurses) don't think that they are influenced by drug company payments, they do think that most of their colleagues *are* influenced. Many other professions aren't permitted to have financial relationships with groups that may influence their opinions, but we allow it in the medical profession.

What's more, the way these conflicts are dealt with is less than optimal. In academia (journals, conferences) and in clinical practice, they are dealt with by stipulating that conflicts of interest must be *declared*. The idea behind this is that the audience or patients can judge the potential effect of any conflict for themselves. The problem is that people don't judge their doctors negatively for these conflicts because they trust doctors. Declarations of conflicts are a poor substitute for *removal* of conflicts, and arguably a waste of time.

There's also evidence that conflicts of interest impact the treatment guidelines generated by expert panels. In a study of two independently produced practice guidelines for a specific blood condition, the guideline produced by panel members with financial ties to industry made recommendations that were more likely to favour the drugs made by those industry ties than the guideline written by experts selected for their independence. Unfortunately, although truly independent expert panels are ideal because they remove this bias towards treatment, they're difficult to achieve because of the rarity of non-conflicted experts in many fields.

The more you do, the more you get paid

There's evidence that financial incentives outside industry also influence practice. Practice can vary depending on how the doctor is paid. Doctors in the United States are paid per procedure, whereas doctors in many other countries, such as the United Kingdom, are salaried (paid a regular wage, regardless of how many procedures they perform). This is one explanation for the much higher rates of spinal fusion and many other procedures in the United States than in the United Kingdom. Australia provides a unique environment to examine this problem because it has a two-tiered system: everyone is covered with universal health care provided by the government, and about half of the population also have private insurance. The rates of spinal fusion surgery in the private sector (where doctors are paid much more to operate than in the public sector) are far higher than in the public sector. This private–public difference in spinal surgery is also far greater than the difference for procedures that are less susceptible to 'surgeon preference', such as hip replacement. While the rate of hip replacements in private hospitals is about twice that in public hospitals, for spinal fusion the difference is about tenfold.

Private hospital profits are roughly proportional to the number of patients who pass through their doors. They've been known to attack research and researchers suggesting that any of their services are unnecessary, and they will use doctors to pen the letters. This is exactly what happened after one of our research institutes published research showing that keeping knee replacement patients in hospital for rehabilitation for a week or more after their surgery was no better for them than simply sending them home, and it cost a lot more.

In some hospitals and for some surgeons, 100 per cent of knee replacement patients are referred to inpatient rehabilitation for about a week. This provides significant income for the hospital and treating rehabilitation doctors, but no benefit for patients who could be going home instead. The Private Hospital Association, which stood to lose a major source of income (inpatient rehabilitation), sent out a media release (signed by a rehabilitation specialist and an orthopaedic surgeon) accusing the research of being 'a ploy by insurers', 'dangerous' and adding that it 'could have disastrous consequences for many Australians'. It should be noted that the research wasn't a one-off: it's well accepted that routine inpatient rehabilitation provides no benefit for patients who can be cared for at home.

The use of procedures varies between doctors, often because of uncertainty regarding their effectiveness or a lack of supporting evidence. In other words, it may not work but some surgeons believe it does, and the more they get paid, the more likely they are to believe it works. Previous research has put the increase in surgery rates from 'fee-for-service' payments at about 80 per cent more than the rates among salaried doctors. Internationally, there have been calls to dismantle fee-for-service payment systems and instead focus on payment for health outcomes rather than the specific treatments provided.

Perhaps the most concerning correlation between financial gain and doctors' rates of prescribing, consulting and operating occurs when doctors own the hospital in which they work. The profit from owning a private hospital increases with turnover, and surgeons who own and work in a hospital have significant control over that turnover. Surgeons who own hospitals are more likely to refer patients for surgery, and they don't always declare this conflict to their patients.

Of course, this problem also applies to non-surgical specialists and primary care providers. Self-referral, the practice of referring patients for tests to facilities in which the doctor or their partners have a financial interest, is a particular issue for imaging tests. The cost of unnecessary self-referred imaging in the United States in 2004 was conservatively estimated to be US$16 billion. One US study reported that the greatest predictor of a patient being referred for an X-ray was whether the referrer owned the machine, while another found that being cared for by a physician who practised self-referral for imaging studies could substantially increase the likelihood of have an imaging test. Not only is this care costly, but there's also consistent evidence of overtesting, as indicated by a higher rate of negative findings in self-referred imaging than in imaging requested by doctors without self-interests.

If we're interested in health as the outcome of health care, then profiting from delivering that care is a flawed model, because it will result in lots of health care without necessarily affecting health. In a way, health care (tests and treatments) has become the surrogate outcome for health.

Regardless of external financial influences such as health industry sponsorship and how a doctor's income is structured, doctors in private practice do have other financial pressures. They have to run a business, and to do that responsibly they need to cover their costs, which can be considerable. Apart from the usual costs of running a practice (rent, staff, supplies, and so on) doctors also have to pay for their own continuing education and their medical defence insurance, which is often many tens of thousands of dollars each year. Particularly in the United States, but increasingly in other countries such as Australia, doctors also start practice with massive debt due to the cost of the education needed to obtain their degree in the first place. To cover the debt and the ongoing practice costs, and to make a profit to support themselves and possibly a family, doctors have to earn a lot of money, money that's almost exclusively generated by treating people.

On the surface, paying doctors to treat people makes sense – we generally pay people for services they perform – but often the benefits of those services are immediately tangible and not debatable. If we pay someone to get the dents out of our car, we can immediately see that it's been successful and if it isn't, we might not pay for it. In medicine, the doctor gets paid regardless of the results.

The capitalist model: an example from China

The problem of paying doctors to treat people irrespective of the outcome can be seen in an example from 1980s China. In the move to privatise health services, each health facility was allowed to make a profit, and doctors' incomes were dependent on that profit – an ideal capitalist model. Given the profit available to them from prescribing drugs and ordering expensive tests such as CT and MRI scans, that's what they did. The more drugs they prescribed and tests they ordered, the more they got paid. This led to an expensive, wasteful and often ineffective healthcare system.

Many patients weren't helped and many were harmed. Although the Chinese government is now trying to untangle the mess, it has left a culture where patients perceive drug prescription and high-cost tests as a necessary component of good care, and often refuse to leave a consultation without multiple prescriptions. It's a classic and large-scale example of the problem with a purely profit-driven healthcare model that rewards *activity*, not health.

* * *

Treating numbers appeals to our desire to be in control. Measuring a number, no matter how unreliable or meaningless that number may be, and using that number to guide treatment, gives both doctor and patient a feeling of control and order. It's a process that can be monitored and seemingly judged as successful or not. Yet by focusing too much on the numbers and not the patient, doctors have fallen into the trap the Oath warns against.

The solution to this is easier than for many of the other problems described in this book. We need to improve the science, but the solution can be as simple as avoiding the use of surrogate outcomes where possible and only targeting outcomes that are *directly* relevant to a person's wellbeing. In some cases, surrogate outcomes may be used, but only if they are known to be very closely related to the important outcomes, or if longer-term follow-up also includes the important outcomes.

Doctors must also recognise their biases and their attraction to treating the numbers. They need to thoroughly evaluate the evidence for treating the number or the scan. This goes for patients and those funding health care as well. If we're not making people live longer or happier lives (i.e. improving quantity and/or quality of life), we're wasting our time. If we don't know whether we are, we need to find out by calling for the evidence and getting it *before* we risk harming people and before we spend money on new treatments. We also need to recognise the drivers of this behaviour, such as financial incentives. The manufacturers and providers of the tests and treatments are too biased to make the rules about who gets treated for what. Those decisions should be made objectively, by non-conflicted independent experts.

8

Prevention

Hippocratic Oath: I will prevent disease whenever I can,
for prevention is preferable to cure.

'If we could give every individual the right amount of
nourishment and exercise, not too little and not too much,
we would have found the safest way to health'
– attributed to Hippocrates

'He who cures a disease may be the skillfullest,
but he that prevents it is the safest physician'
– Thomas Fuller, 17th–18th century English physician

It's hard to argue with the maxim that prevention is better than cure. But the current focus among doctors on early detection of existing disease and on late individualised treatments has diverted attention away from the oath to 'prevent disease' where possible. In contrast to screening, which aims to detect and treat disease before the patient develops symptoms in order to avoid severe disease or death, prevention aims to stop diseases from occurring in the first place.

Chronic respiratory disease (usually from long-term smoking) is a good example of the bias towards screening over true prevention. Groups of expert doctors, often sponsored by drug companies, have produced recommendations that support detecting chronic respiratory disease early and treating it with drugs. This is despite the fact that drug treatment does almost nothing for chronic respiratory disease, even if it's detected early. In fact, the only treatment that changes the course of disease and lowers the risk of death is to stop smoking, and the disease is preventable if smoking is stopped early or never taken up. The effort to produce such guidelines, to set up programs to detect these patients early, and to treat them with largely ineffective treatments is time that would be better spent joining the doctors who are working to prevent (and treat) the condition through smoking prevention and quitting programs.

Public health: the most effective prevention

Life expectancy has roughly doubled, from around 40 to 80 years, since the mid-1800s. It's well established that this improvement has been largely due to public health (e.g. clean water, sanitation), industry (e.g. food production, preservation and transport), politics (fewer wars) and social changes (e.g. education, welfare, housing, and regulations concerning work safety, and air and food quality). It may be well established, but it is not well *known*.

In one US survey, researchers found that people rarely attribute the increase in life expectancy to public health or social change. In fact, only 2 per cent of respondents thought that sanitation was the most important contributor. They attributed only around 20 per cent of the improvement in life expectancy to public health and lifestyle changes. They believed that, even with improvements in sanitation, food supply, income and education, without modern medicine the current life expectancy would only be 47 years – not much more than it was 200 years ago. The US Centers for Disease Control has concluded the opposite. Based on research evidence, it credited about 80 per cent of the improvements in life expectancy (i.e. 25 of the 30 years our lives have been extended by in the 20th century alone) to public health measures. And this was taking into account the fact that during this period, modern medicine, antibiotics and safe surgery have blossomed.

There's no doubt that life expectancy has risen beyond most people's expectations, and many have been keen to attribute that to medicine. But medical care provided to individuals, including cancer treatments, antibiotics and insulin for people with diabetes, to give just a few examples, has contributed only a *fraction* to the improvement in life expectancy.

Falling numbers of deaths from heart attacks

Take heart attacks, for example. They were once one of the biggest causes of death, but since about the 1970s, the number of deaths from heart attacks has fallen consistently. Many people today would attribute that to modern medical interventions such as coronary artery bypass surgery and stenting. But as we have seen, most stenting doesn't reduce deaths, and there is little difference in mortality after bypass surgery compared with stenting. Furthermore, the decline in deaths from heart attacks started before these treatments became widely available.

So what has caused the decline in cardiac deaths? Most of the decrease can be attributed to social or lifestyle changes: less smoking, better diets and more exercise.

Falling numbers of deaths from infectious diseases

The biggest drop in deaths over the last 150–200 years is due to a decline in dying from infectious diseases. In the 1800s one of, if not *the*, biggest cause of death was tuberculosis (also known as TB or consumption), an infection now treatable with antibiotics. Most people would attribute the rarity of tuberculosis these days to medical treatment with antibiotics, but nearly all of the reduction in deaths from this disease has been due to improvements in sanitation and nutrition. By the time antibiotics were even discovered for tuberculosis, the death rate had already fallen by about 90 per cent and was still falling.

Vaccines have been very successful in some areas, notably for smallpox, which has been eradicated by a vaccine. While these are administered to individuals (unlike, say, water fluoridation), they are usually given to whole populations, on a mass scale. In Australia, the important vaccines are mandated – you have to make an effort *not* to have them. We would argue that vaccines fall outside individual modern medical care: they're not something you seek out or something given in response to a complaint – the *default* is to vaccinate. But even vaccines don't compete with food, water, shelter and safety when it comes to their effect on life expectancy. The rates of typhus, cholera, whooping cough, scarlet fever, influenza and measles had all fallen dramatically before vaccines for them were ever introduced. Almost all of the decline in these once common diseases was due to public health measures.

COVID-19

As the COVID outbreak unfolded, we became accustomed to listening to the experts – the infectious disease specialists and the epidemiologists – and we're all now familiar with the need to 'flatten the curve' to prevent overwhelming hospitals and intensive care units. Throughout the pandemic, the experts, and even some amateurs, have crunched the numbers to determine when restrictions are necessary and when it might be safe to ease them, as well as how to ease the restrictions. In some ways, the public have had a crash course in the science of medicine. Many people now even know what an epidemiologist is, and the crucial role they've been playing in stemming the pandemic.

We have lived experience of the scientific gains made during this pandemic. Initial expert advice was based upon what we already knew from previous epidemics, but new information emerged rapidly, sometimes changing the advice, and we had to learn to adapt. Based upon how we know viruses spread, including the ones that cause the common cold (which can spread through the air and from touching contaminated objects), the initial emphasis was on washing hands, disinfecting surfaces and avoiding touching your face. While these precautions are still worthwhile, and contributed to a drop in cold and flu cases, we now know that the SARS-CoV-2 virus that causes COVID-19 spreads primarily by being expelled in the air rather than from contaminated surfaces. Some small particles can persist in the air for a long time, particularly indoors and where there is poor ventilation.

Initially there was conflicting advice about masks, with experts divided on their value. There were also concerns that it would make people complacent about social distancing as well as worsen shortages of personal protective equipment for health professionals and others who really needed them. There's no longer any doubt, however, that the use of masks reduces the spread of virus in aerosol particles and at least partially protects people who wear them.

We also now understand what happens when preventive measures fall short, having now seen many local examples, not to mention the inadequacies of health care that have been exposed in the aged-care sector. We can also be thankful that in Australia the pandemic response has largely been driven by science and not politics. As a recent article in the *Scientific American* stated, 'The most important public health measure during a pandemic of a disease with no cure or vaccine – as many countries around the world that have controlled the virus have shown – is to help experts share clear, trustworthy, accurate, actionable information based on the best evidence. Spreading lies has spread the disease'.

The pandemic sparked a huge international research effort directed towards finding effective and safe vaccines, as well as effective treatments. But even without vaccines and effective treatments, many countries, particularly in East Asia and Australia and New Zealand, were able to drastically minimise the spread and the number of deaths through public health measures that prevented people from getting the disease, reducing the harm from the virus far more than any treatment to date.

Preventing diseases due to smoking

Smoking contributes to about 9 per cent of all deaths worldwide. Significant gains in the prevention of tobacco-related disease have been made in some countries, and especially here in Australia, but this only came about after decades of dedicated work from a small group of concerned clinicians and researchers. This group was pushing against an industry that didn't want to prevent the diseases and a government that didn't want to lose the associated income from smokers. In the battle against smoking, in fact, it was the harm to third parties (from passive smoking) that made it possible to pass so many anti-smoking laws. This raises questions about society's priorities in protecting people from harm that arises from their own actions, seen as a personal responsibility, versus harm that arises from others, seen as a societal responsibility.

In other countries, however, smoking rates are increasing. China has one of the highest smoking rates in the world, particularly among men, most of whom smoke. Anti-smoking laws exist but are rarely enforced. Given that the tobacco industry accounts for around 10 per cent of government revenue, you can see at least one reason why this might be the case. The problem isn't helped by the fact that about half of all male doctors in China smoke.

Smoking in China is expected to be responsible for hundreds of millions of deaths. Given that half of all smokers will die of a smoking-related disease, this means that at least a quarter of all men in China will die of a smoking-related disease. The detection and treatment of smoking-related conditions such as heart disease, vascular disease and lung cancer will have an unimaginable cost and little effect, especially compared to measures to prevent smoking.

Smoking rates in many countries such as Australia and the United States have at least halved since the 1980s. This is disease prevention on a massive scale, especially compared to many of the other kinds of disease prevention proposed by doctors.

The medical industry and prevention

While many doctors are actively trying to prevent disease in effective ways, by targeting the big-ticket items like smoking, alcohol and obesity, others have predominantly put their efforts into treating the conditions associated with these, often seeing prevention as futile. In other instances the medical industry backs prevention initiatives, but for dubious reasons. The overemphasis on early detection programs that don't provide true prevention stands in contrast to the medical industry's lack of support for 'real' prevention programs that arguably have a larger impact on the health of individuals and society as a whole. Some of the greatest contributors to the societal burden of disease, including death and disability, come from preventable conditions such as obesity and the use of legal drugs, largely alcohol and tobacco, but also drugs such as opioids.

Disease 'awareness' initiatives

These days, the public face of 'prevention' programs often comes in the form of disease 'awareness' programs, which aim to increase the treatment of existing conditions rather than preventing them in the first place. A particular problem is programs that tie into drug treatments and procedures that reward those in the medical industry. This is because much of the support for these initiatives comes from the medical industry (doctors, pharma, hospital owners, device manufacturers and so on). The backing can be direct, through financial support or lobbying, or indirect through the support of consumer organisations and research. The list of conditions that have been subject to these types of initiatives is long, but includes sexual dysfunction, binge eating disorder, attention deficit hyperactivity disorder (ADHD), social anxiety, restless leg syndrome, dry eye, depression and osteoporosis.

Raising awareness of spinal fractures from osteoporosis

One illustration of the way industry combines with advocacy groups to spin misleading messages was highlighted in August 2018, when healthnewsreview.org published an article about an emailed announcement from a public relations company. In preparation for World Osteoporosis Day (20 August), two US national advocacy groups, the National Osteoporosis Foundation and the National Bone Health Alliance, had joined forces with Medtronic, the largest medical device company in the world, to 'raise awareness' for what they considered to be an underdiagnosed problem – spinal fractures due to osteoporosis.

They were promoting a treatment called kyphoplasty, a procedure not unlike vertebroplasty (see chapter 2), in which Medtronic happens to be highly invested. Rather than just injecting the fractured vertebra with cement, a balloon is inflated within the fractured vertebra first, purportedly to maintain the height of the spine. In the announcement, they used an example to suggest that this procedure will give people their lives back and that it is the only alternative to a life of opioids and excruciating pain. The problem, however, is that most spinal fractures heal quickly and only require temporary pain relief. Furthermore, the efficacy of kyphoplasty is unproven. Unlike vertebroplasty, it hasn't yet been the subject of any high-quality trials that compare it to placebo, although it seems to work (or not work) about the same as vertebroplasty. Not only were both advocacy groups conflicted by financial relationships with Medtronic, but the doctor who featured in the promotional materials was also similarly conflicted.

Preventing diseases due to alcohol

One area of disease prevention that hasn't been adequately addressed in many societies is alcohol consumption. Alcohol contributes to around 3 per cent of all deaths (about a third the rate of death from smoking) and around 4 per cent of all the years lost due to disability (about the same as smoking, because smoking kills more than it disables). In other words, alcohol isn't as big a killer as smoking, but it's just as bad when it comes to harmful effects on people's lives and on society. Alcohol is linked to the development of many cancers, liver disease, disease of the pancreas, gastric bleeding, mental health issues, violence, memory loss, diminished sexual function, road trauma, birth defects, osteoporosis and many other conditions.

Yet there's a paucity of prevention strategies to reduce harm from alcohol consumption. How much of this is due to the influence of industry – not just the producers of alcoholic drinks but many other industries such as retail and service – and how much is due to cultural resistance? It's hard to tell, because the acceptability of alcohol remains high, whereas the acceptability of smoking has changed considerably in many cultures. Needless to say, there's a lot of money to be made in the business of alcohol, including by governments.

Preventing obesity-related illness

Obesity is associated with an increased risk of early death, as well as with conditions that have a major impact on quality of life and disability, including type 2 diabetes, osteoarthritis, heart disease, liver disease, kidney disease and certain cancers. While there are many contributors to obesity, including personal decisions and local cultural factors, our current 'food environment' – the food choices we make and the relative costs of those choices – is contributing to obesity. And that environment is largely controlled by the food producers and marketers.

Our food environment pushes energy-dense (more calories per bite) foods in many ways, by making them more available, more appealing and cheaper. And like the tobacco industry, the food industry deflects the blame, pointing to lack of exercise rather than the intake of calories as the cause of the obesity problem. It also lobbies governments to protect their business, which is to sell as much product as possible at the highest price possible to as many people as they can.

On the surface, it appears to be a lot easier to treat someone who has type 2 diabetes or cardiovascular disease with drugs rather than try to help them lose weight. This is despite the fact that losing weight can dramatically alter the severity and outcomes of these chronic diseases. For many of these diseases, weight loss will improve the condition so much that drugs and other treatments will no longer be necessary. Weight loss can cause adult-onset diabetes to literally disappear, and therefore reduce all the associated conditions that go along with that diagnosis (infections, vascular disease, heart attacks, kidney failure and blindness, for example), yet we tend to just go on treating each condition without emphasising the benefits of weight loss. The patients, too, often want a quick fix, but sometimes that's because the benefits and opportunities to lose weight aren't emphasised by their doctors.

The problem is that the effort needed in getting individual patients to quit smoking, cut down on drinking or to lose weight is considerable and often unrewarding, and the incentives are low. The medical industry remains disease-focused and procedure-focused. This is reflected in the fact that so much effort and promotion has been put into treating the condition with surgery rather than preventing it in the first place. Obesity surgery is more expensive, riskier and less beneficial than obesity prevention.

Treating obesity to prevent diseases is hard, but the smarter approach would be changing culture and regulations to prevent obesity, which would make treatment unnecessary for many. By preventing the root cause leading to so many other conditions, we would be able to prevent a lot more deaths and suffering. A change in culture and regulations around smoking has had a huge impact on health. We can do the same thing with the overuse of alcohol and with the rising obesity epidemic.

There are communities and societies where this has been achieved. Even within modern cities, there are regions of high obesity and regions where it's rare. Paradoxically, the geographic distribution of these regions parallels the distribution of socioeconomic status: the richer people are, the less obese they are. In a way this is perhaps the opposite of we would expect from history, when obesity was a sign of wealth (of being able to afford food).

The current association between lower socioeconomic status and obesity has several likely causes. Firstly, high-energy food such as fast food and sweetened drinks are cheap, often really cheap. But more than that, they taste good because we evolved when high-energy foods were much less available than they are today. This meant that our intake was lower, and we tended to fill up when we could because we were never sure when the next meal might come along. The lack of availability also meant that we burned a lot of energy getting the food in the first place.

The other reason behind the lack of obesity seen in higher socioeconomic areas is education. People with higher education know that obesity is bad, and that fitness is good, and they can 'afford' the time to exercise and to buy (more expensive) healthier food.

So should doctors be advocating a better economy to prevent disease? Yes and no. While it's true that within many countries, people with higher socioeconomic status are less likely to be obese (or to smoke), there are still cultures where obesity isn't such a problem, regardless of socioeconomic status. There's considerable variation in obesity rates between countries that can't be explained by their economic differences. For example, Japan, South Korea and Italy have the lowest rates of obesity compared to other OECD countries, and the United States and Mexico have the highest. Some of the richest countries in the world, like Norway, Singapore and Switzerland, have very low rates of obesity, yet other rich countries such as the United States, Australia and Germany (which shares a border with Switzerland) have some of the most obese. At the other end of the spectrum, many Pacific island nations (with lower socioeconomic status) have the highest rates of obesity, while other low-income countries, such as Sri Lanka and Indonesia, have some of the lowest obesity rates in the world. These examples show that significant local cultural factors can interact with socioeconomic factors.

Changing the culture to reduce obesity is a big task, and involves such diverse groups as governments, non-government organisations, town planners, business, advertisers and individual role models, but it also involves doctors. The campaign against smoking involved doctors, and doctors are well placed to play an influential role in any push against obesity and alcohol. If they wish to truly live up to their oath to prevent disease, this is where the greatest good can be done.

Obesity prevention can be achieved by governments, using methods adopted from tobacco control, by changing laws concerning taxation of energy-dense food, packaging and advertising, urban planning (encouraging exercise), school education programs and zoning regulations (for example, many hospitals are no longer allowed to carry sweetened drinks and unhealthy snacks in their shops or vending machines).

Preventing back pain

In contrast to the many hundreds of studies assessing *treatments* for low back pain (see chapter 5), very few have looked at ways of preventing back pain in the first place – primary prevention. One reason may be that it's hard to find people who have never experienced back pain. Most of the prevention trials have included adults who have had back pain already and the treatment in question is trying to prevent it recurring – secondary prevention.

Most of the strategies touted to prevent back pain, such as softer or firmer mattresses, back supports and belts, shoe insoles and ergonomic furniture, have either been proven ineffective or are poorly studied. Low back pain is a common problem in the workplace and a common cause of sick leave, and yet attempts to prevent low back pain in the workplace have been largely unsuccessful. Strategies such as workplace education, no-lift policies and ergonomic interventions are ineffective. Businesses have used education about lifting materials and assistive devices in an attempt to minimise low back pain. But a high-quality review of lifting advice and assistive devices concluded that they don't prevent back pain or back-pain-related disability.

Just about the only strategy that has some evidence to support it is exercise, with or without education. These trials were, however, all secondary-prevention trials, performed in unusual study populations such as military personnel, and the exercise regimes were quite intensive. Whether or not these results would translate to the general population is unclear.

Where are the doctors in all this?

If the medical community were to truly live up to their oath to prevent disease, they would spend less time on low-value detection programs and promotion of end-stage treatments, and more time targeting smoking, alcohol and obesity at both an individual and societal level.

A government-supported advertising program to change the 'sun' culture in Australia and encourage protection measures has resulted in a significant decrease in skin cancers and associated deaths. Other government initiatives in the fields of obesity and alcohol exist, but much more can be done. And there's a place for doctors to lead this.

We consider the main problem with doctors getting involved in prevention is that disease treatment fits much better into a business model for medicine. Prevention is done on a large scale, something often best left to governments. But even for governments, it might appear easier to pay for each treatment needed as a result of obesity – lifetime diabetes care, renal dialysis, foot ulcer care, cardiac stenting, joint replacement and gastric bypass surgery – than to prevent it in the first place. It's hard to fund a model based on dietary intake and exercise; it's much easier to fund procedures. The medical business favours late-stage treatment over prevention, and the hospital owners, doctors, and drug and device manufacturers and distributors all benefit from it. Even for the insurers, this type of care is easier to predict and set premiums for than disease prevention.

As with many of the other problems addressed in this book, one solution is to redesign the medical system away from addressing disease towards improving health. An easier solution would be to divert money away from ineffective screening programs towards effective prevention programs, such as the anti-smoking programs introduced in some countries. We should be careful, however, not to introduce large-scale 'real' prevention programs for problems such as smoking and obesity without proper evaluation by conducting rigorous large-scale studies.

* * *

Real prevention of disease using large-scale public health measures, including legal controls, taxes and advertising, has led to massive improvements in health over the past few centuries. More recently this has prevented millions of deaths from heart disease, lung cancer and many other cancers. Large-scale public health measures, where they were adhered to, also prevented thousands if not millions of deaths from COVID-19.

Preventive programs are needed today due to the massive but preventable health impacts of our current lifestyle. Doctors hold a unique position in society to drive this change, as they have done with tobacco control.

9
Medicalising normal

Hippocratic Oath: I will remember that I remain a member of society, with special obligations to all my fellow human beings, those of sound mind and body as well as the infirm.

'The greatest medicine of all is teaching people how not to need it'
– attributed to Hippocrates

'Medical science is making such remarkable progress that soon none of us will be well'
– attributed to Aldous Huxley

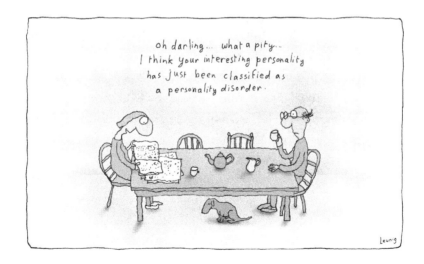

Which of the following would you class a disease and which as normal: deafness, attention deficit hyperactivity disorder (ADHD), alcoholism, erectile dysfunction, tension headache, irritable bowel syndrome, high cholesterol, chronic fatigue syndrome, menopause, obesity? In a survey conducted in 2010, laypeople, doctors, nurses and members of parliament in Australia were asked to rate a series of 60 conditions as diseases or normal. The researchers deliberately included a spectrum of conditions. At one end, nearly everybody 'strongly agreed' that breast cancer and pneumonia, for example, are diseases, and, at the other end, nearly everybody agreed that ageing and homosexuality aren't diseases. What was interesting was where there was disagreement. Between the two ends of the spectrum were conditions like those we listed at the beginning of this paragraph.

To further demonstrate the blurring of the line between normal and disease, in a similar study participants were more likely to label conditions as diseases if medical terminology was used. For example, erectile dysfunction and impotence are two labels for exactly the same condition, but in this study erectile dysfunction, the more medical or technical term, was considered a disease but impotence wasn't. Similarly, hypertension was considered a disease but high blood pressure, which is exactly the same thing, wasn't.

As we saw in chapter 5, the processes by which normal human conditions come to be defined and treated as medical conditions is termed 'medicalisation'. Medicalisation isn't *inherently* bad, but the question is whether it results in a *net* good, and if there's actually anything to be gained by medicalising 'normal'?

This chapter's pledge in the Hippocratic Oath is a reminder to doctors that they have a special obligation to ensure they're not harming their fellow human beings who are not *truly* infirm – 'those of sound mind and body' or, more specifically, those who *feel* well.

To medicalise or not to medicalise?

Premenstrual dysmorphic disorder (PMDD) became an officially recognised medical diagnosis in 2012 when it made it into the *DSM*. PMDD could be considered a 'normal' predicament of life in that it affects 3–8 per cent of menstruating women, but the diagnosis refers to a severe and disabling form of premenstrual syndrome that can have a range of distressing mental and physical effects. The mental effects can include marked mood swings, irritability, anger, depression and anxiety, as well as feeling overwhelmed or out of control. Some women become suicidal – one study found 15 per cent of women with the condition had attempted suicide – and many succeed. The symptoms occur during the week before menstruation and disappear at its onset. The cause isn't established, but experts consider that it's likely due to a combination of increased sensitivity to fluctuating levels of the reproductive hormones, genetic predisposition and environmental stress.

The 'medicalisation' of this disorder came as a relief for Rachelle. Although she had never sought care, it finally explained her longstanding symptoms (and that of some of her patients), and helped allay her guilt for what she has put those close to her through at times over many years. That's just one person for whom the label has been helpful. A better understanding of the biological processes that underlie the disorder could also result in better treatment for those who are severely afflicted, and result in better outcomes including less self-harm.

Yet there's still a risk of medicalising PMDD to the point of causing net harm. PMDD is at the severe end of the premenstrual syndrome spectrum, but what if the criteria were broadened to include more menstruating women with milder symptoms? According to a 2019 BBC *Future* article by Christine Ro, there has been some criticism of the links between the *DSM* subcommittee members who made the decision to recognise PMDD and pharma companies, amid concerns that the condition would be overmedicalised for profit. Ro also noted that 'some sceptics are nervous about attaching another label to women that presents them as irrational'.

The bottom line is that medicalisation cannot simply be *assumed* to be good (or bad). Its benefits are often overestimated, while its harms are underestimated. In this chapter we're primarily concerned with medicalisation that leads to overdiagnosis – the harmful labelling as diseased of normal people without risk factors or true disease. As for PMDD, in some circumstances labelling may be helpful for simply describing a set of symptoms, even without specific treatment. It can be reassuring, and a way of acknowledging suffering and confirming the reality of symptoms. On the other hand, some medical labels serve no useful purpose and may be disconnected from any identifiable pathological process or disease. When the diagnosis becomes embedded in a disease–illness paradigm, it can trigger the doctor's desire to treat, regardless of the likelihood of benefit.

Diagnosing people with 'normal' complaints

It can be difficult to decide what symptoms, or degree of symptoms, should be considered 'normal'. Should people who are sad be diagnosed with depression, or is it normal? Are shy people or autistic people part of a normal spectrum? When does back pain or a change in bowel habits go beyond normal?

Depression

The debate over the diagnosis of depression has been going on for some time and is made harder because it's a very subjective condition with a lot of contributing factors and a wide spectrum of severity and chronicity. At one end of the spectrum, it's normal to feel sad if something bad happens to you like losing a loved one

– it's a normal reaction and is usually self-limiting. Most people wouldn't call that depression, yet people in that situation still get treated with antidepressant medication. At the other end of the spectrum is 'major' depression, a severe form of depression that goes far beyond what would normally be classed as a normal reaction. Between these two extremes are a lot of people, people who could be treated as 'normal' or as having a medical condition that requires medical treatment.

The medicalisation of depression has been very successful – successful in that many people who don't feel happy have been medicalised and treated, not because they got better. Antidepressants make up some of the most commonly prescribed medications in the world (around one in eight adults in Australia). Many of them are blockbuster drugs, drawing in billions in revenue each year, yet some of the most popular antidepressants either don't work at all, or don't work for the majority of people who take them. And they have harmful psychological and physical effects.

The overdiagnosis and overtreatment of depression is well documented: how drug companies have made ineffective drugs look effective by only publishing the positive studies and holding back the negative ones; how the drugs have been used for teenagers despite good evidence of lack of effectiveness and an increased risk of suicidal thoughts in that age group; and the role of industry relations among doctors involved in the panels that decide on the diagnostic criteria.

But the relevance of overdiagnosis to this chapter is not how unscrupulous the drug companies have been, but whether the person who is depressed benefits from being medicalised. The test of whether medicalising something is good or bad lies in the evidence, not in the intention. Yet doctors tend to judge themselves on their intentions, not on an objective evaluation of the consequences of their actions. It has been estimated that the majority of people who have been treated for depression have been overdiagnosed and overtreated – the *majority* of one of the most common diagnoses on the planet. Costs aside, that's a lot of psychological harm from being labelled and a lot of physical harm from the ill effects of the medications.

One of the signs of possible overdiagnosis is when the incidence of the disease increases over time, which is certainly the case with depression. It's unlikely that people are getting sadder over years and decades; it's more likely that the bar is being lowered. That means we're taking people who used to be considered normal and labelling them as abnormal. That's when the alarm bells should ring and we should ask ourselves whether this is good for those diagnosed. When the first antidepressant drug was developed, the drug company didn't think there was a market for it. Now, according to national surveys, more than 13 per cent of all US adults have used antidepressant medication in the last 30 days; for women over 60, it's about a quarter. Australian data shows that 15 per cent of all adults received an antidepressant prescription in the past year, one of the highest rates internationally.

Autism

Autism, also called autism spectrum disorder, describes a spectrum of disease that merges with normal somewhere. In diagnosing it we're attempting to help those who are slightly different, but in our eagerness to help, we're sometimes causing unseen and unmeasured harm.

There is an argument in the field of autism that people with this condition should be considered part of the spectrum of normal, not part of the spectrum of disease – that while autistic people are different from the 'average', they're still part of what we should consider normal. Let's consider the benefits of treating autism as normal.

Many people with autism wish to be treated as equal members of society, not as impaired. They reject the notion that they're something 'other'. They consider themselves no more different than many other people with non-average physical and psychological attributes. Most people with autism live and work in the community, and many around them don't even know they have it. Where's the benefit in the label for the majority? Some people with autism have learning disabilities, but this problem can be identified and treated separately. What does the *additional* diagnosis of autism add for the person with a learning disability?

Much of the push to label autism as a disease has come from the idea that medication may help, and the research that has pushed this line has largely been funded by those most likely to profit from drug sales.

Although no genetic basis has been found for autism, even in conditions where there is a clear genetic basis, the labelling has not always been helpful. In Down syndrome, for example, there's a long history of hurtful and dehumanising labelling. For them, being labelled as abnormal and mentally disordered only has negative effects, and creates a sense of 'otherness' that contributes to their social separation. People have been labelled abnormal in the past, only to be considered normal in more 'enlightened' times. At the moment, autism is framed as a deficit, disability, disorder and impairment – negative words that make us want to correct (treat) the condition.

Low back pain

As we saw earlier, for a long time, people have coped with common, simple back pain – the condition isn't new, it's just that there was previously no point labelling it. In many indigenous populations, low back pain is still considered a relatively benign part of daily life. It only becomes a medical problem when these populations become exposed to Western health care, where low back pain has been medicalised. Back pain is now entrenched in the disease–

illness paradigm, but medicalising the normal experience of low back pain can lead to significant harms.

For doctors, rather than providing advice and assurance of a likely good outcome, the inclination is to treat. And they have an increasing number of possible, and mostly unproven, treatments at their disposal – surgery, strong painkillers, injections, manipulations, osteopathy, and so on. The use of these treatments varies widely, both between countries and within them. This means you might be treated very differently depending on where you live and who you see. If your doctor uses injections in the spine to treat back pain, for example, that's more than likely what you will be offered. Yet spinal injection treatments are either marginally or no more effective than placebo.

Treating workplace-related low back complaints with surgery also has a bad track record, with high rates of reoperation, dissatisfaction, prolonged opioid use, need for ongoing treatment and failure to return to work. Treatment with opioids alone is no better. A study recently completed by one of Rachelle's PhD students, Michael Di Donato, found a disturbingly high use of opioids among Australian workers with low back pain who had been off work with an accepted worker's compensation claim. One-third had received at least one opioid prescription, and their use was associated with significantly longer time off work. People prescribed moderate to high amounts of opioids over the longer term had a median time off work approaching two and a half years (126 weeks) compared with 7.1 weeks in those who weren't prescribed them, and about 31 weeks in those who were only prescribed a limited amount for a short time.

Irritable bowel syndrome

Irritable bowel syndrome (IBS) is the most common gastrointestinal diagnosis, but it's not exactly clear what it is. IBS has no formal diagnostic test or clear cause, and the symptoms can be anything from vague abdominal pain to altered bowel habit. But what is a normal bowel habit? The criteria for this disease include 'visceral hypersensitivity' which could mean complaining too much about your stomach. The treatment emphasises addressing psychosocial factors, which means there's a little more to IBS than just the gut.

IBS is to the gastroenterologist as back pain is to the orthopaedic surgeon, fibromyalgia to the rheumatologist, headache to the neurologist, and so on. The diagnosis is often unclear and often changes, there's no clear theory regarding the cause, psychosocial factors are often implicated, there's a wide variation in the degree of distress people are in, and there are lots of treatments with questionable effectiveness.

The bottom line here is that what constitutes normal for bowel discomfort and regularity varies a lot. Some people probably satisfy the criteria for IBS but are never diagnosed because, if they are not sufficiently worried or concerned, they never seek an opinion – whereas those with identical symptoms and signs who consult a gastroenterologist get diagnosed with IBS.

A diagnosis of IBS entails the same problems as the other diagnoses we have discussed. Some people receive treatment that makes them feel better, but they may have felt better without the label, and without the treatment. Many who are labelled are no better off for being 'diagnosed' and may be harmed from attempted treatments.

Attention deficit hyperactivity disorder

ADHD is the most diagnosed condition of childhood and is now diagnosed in adults. The idea that this is either not a real disease or, at best, a highly overdiagnosed one is supported by studies that show huge variations in the rate of diagnosis and treatment over time, among certain age and gender groups, and between geographic regions where the rate of diagnosis likely reflects the differing opinions of local practitioners rather than any difference in the people who live there.

In Australia, the variation in prescribing rates per capita between the highest and lowest geographic regions for ADHD drugs is a factor of 75. Either children in some regions are being undertreated, or kids in other regions are being overtreated, or both. In classrooms, where about 10 per cent of children may be diagnosed with ADHD, one of the strongest predictors of the diagnosis is a child's date of birth: younger children within a classroom are more likely to be diagnosed. Immaturity is being labelled as a mental disease.

Let's put aside the debate about whether it's a true disease or a social construction labelling a spectrum of 'normal' as a disease, and the fact that it has huge support from the drug industry through lobby groups, sponsored consumer organisations, doctors, academics and sponsored research. Let's accept the fact that there's something noticeably different about people who are diagnosed with ADHD, despite no blood test or scan distinguishing it from 'normal'. Firstly, being different or behaving differently is not necessarily caused by a disease. How 'different' from normal does a person have to be before they're not normal? The current criteria for ADHD from different sources vary so widely that this question has not been clearly answered.

It's also unlikely that ADHD sprang out of nowhere. There were probably a lot of people around exhibiting similar behaviours before it was labelled a disease. What happened to them in the past? This has led to accusations that ADHD wasn't discovered, but invented. Practitioners develop theories about causes and use the availability of treatments to justify labelling, instead of asking whether labelling someone with ADHD makes their life better. It might do for some, but not all, and the downside of diagnosing and treating ADHD is often not factored in when starting down this path.

Psychiatry has been widely criticised for medicalising normal, and for relying on medications over non-pharmacological therapies. We've already mentioned autism and ADHD, but now grief is working its way into the *DSM* and is being treated with antidepressants. There's evidence that these drugs aren't effective. There's also no definitive high-quality evidence to support grief counselling. Are we helping people by medicalising grief? Clearly, we *want* to help, but good intentions aren't good enough if we don't sufficiently consider the harms that can come from applying these labels.

The problems with medicalisation in psychiatry have been addressed in Allen Frances's book *Saving Normal: An Insider's Revolt Against Out-of-Control Psychiatric Diagnosis, DSM-5, Big Pharma, and the Medicalization of Ordinary Life*. Professor Frances, who headed the task force for the fourth edition of the *DSM*, speaks very strongly about the problems with modern psychiatry and its invasion of normalcy, noting, for example, that half of all Americans qualify for a lifetime diagnosis of a mental disorder. One study estimated that 80 per cent of Americans already met the criteria for a mental disorder by the time they were young adults.

Sarcopenia

Sarcopenia is a new condition that was officially accepted as a 'real' disease with its own International Classification of Diseases code (ICD-10) in 2016. Sarcopenia means 'less' or weak muscles. It's normal to lose muscle strength as we age – from the age of 30, people lose 4–5 per cent of their muscle mass every decade. We all therefore get weaker as we get older and even weaker if we can't or don't exercise. One estimate is that one in three Australians over the age of 60 have sarcopenia. Does it have a specific cause and can it be identified with a specific test? No, but people's belief in the condition has led to all sorts of claims, and with these come treatments.

One of the claims is that sarcopenia is a serious disease because it's linked to mortality: the weaker your muscles, the more likely you are to die or be physically disabled. This correlation may be true, but correlation doesn't mean causation: people who are sick (from almost anything) get weak (i.e. exhibit sarcopenia), and the sickness that caused the weakness may also cause them to die. They didn't die *because* they were weak.

But there are now societies of healthcare practitioners dedicated to the study and treatment of sarcopenia. This would be fine if treating people with simple age-related weakness by giving them exercises, for example, improved their quality of life or longevity, but can't we do that anyway without making up new diseases? The harms from such labelling have not been adequately considered, nor have the harms from proposed medical treatments such as growth hormone, testosterone and other drugs that promote muscle growth. Studies that show that muscle mass and strength can be improved with exercise have been taken as proof of the existence of sarcopenia. We would argue that this may be another example of tooth-fairy science.

Newer drugs for sarcopenia are being developed and studied, but we will remain sceptical of their value unless someone gathers good evidence that they're beneficial and their net benefit outweighs their potential for harm – which is perhaps unlikely when you're fighting against the ageing process.

Menopause

Menopause is another normal part of life that has been overmedicalised. For many years, hormone replacement therapy (HRT) was given routinely for menopause in the belief that this would not only prevent or help symptoms but have other health benefits such as a reduction in heart attacks (which are much more common after menopause). The use of hormone replacement was boosted by labelling the condition as 'hormone deficiency syndrome'.

After the practice became routine, evidence from a large, randomised trial comparing HRT to not taking HRT showed the opposite of what was expected: an *increase* in heart attacks from HRT. Consequently, the routine use of HRT quickly declined. More studies have been done since, and while some women benefit from medical treatment to alleviate symptoms, the point here is that harms were done by our readiness to accept that menopause, an entirely natural phenomenon, was a medical condition that always needed to be treated.

Labelling healthy people with disease

Unnecessarily labelling people who have 'normal' complaints with a diagnosis can lead to harm, but there's at least as much or more potential for harm in labelling healthy people with disease. This can arise from broadening existing disease definitions to include asymptomatic people who would not benefit from the label, or creating new diseases or labels to explain a normal spectrum of people.

Pre-hypertension

Vigorous debate has arisen recently about a decision to lower the threshold at which blood pressure is considered abnormal. This recommendation is aimed at preventing the harms from having hypertension (high blood pressure), but while treating people with very high blood pressure may be helpful, when blood pressure levels are only slightly above normal, the actual risk of blood-pressure-related problems is very low. This means we're declaring *many* more people as diseased, because there's a far greater number of people with near-average blood pressure than with very high blood pressure. But very few (if any) of this large group will benefit from treatment.

While the benefits of diagnosis and treatment fall with every lowering of the upper limit of 'normal' blood pressure, the harms from treatment, including the cost, inconvenience and side effects, stay the same. At some point, the harms will outweigh the benefits, but often we only concentrate on the *potential* for benefit, no matter how slight, without balancing this against the harms, no matter how great.

Blood pressure varies between people, and even the same person's blood pressure can change over short periods. If their blood pressure is clearly high (say, more than 160 systolic, where 120 or lower is defined as 'normal'), treatment, which might include simple lifestyle changes with or without drugs, is recommended and is helpful. But that level of blood pressure only occurs in a small proportion of the population.

The harms from treating people with *mildly* elevated blood pressure are several. Firstly, the very act of labelling people raises stress and anxiety levels. Several studies have found higher rates of work absenteeism among people who have simply been labelled with having high blood pressure compared to those who have no knowledge of their blood pressure, or people with normal blood pressure. Secondly, these people now have a 'condition', a disease or diagnosis they wouldn't otherwise have had. This might impact their ability to obtain health, life and travel insurance. Thirdly, they may be out of pocket for the extra treatment, and if they're not paying for it, other premium payers or the government is. And finally, they may suffer side effects from the drugs used to treat their *mildly* elevated blood pressure.

Over the past few decades, the definition of hypertension has been widened to the point where 40 per cent of all adults now have hypertension or 'pre-hypertension'. More than half of 45–75-year-olds now satisfy the definition of abnormally high blood pressure. But if the definition of 'abnormal' includes more than half the population – that is, outnumbering 'normal' people – it suggests we have a problem.

This would be acceptable if the diagnosis carried a downstream benefit, such as reduced mortality or reduced cardiovascular disease as a result of increased treatment, but it doesn't. There's no benefit to the individual or to society in treating well people who have been diagnosed with pre-hypertension. But that hasn't stopped doctors from treating them.

A review of trials of treating blood pressure using the new definitions showed no benefit and an increase in adverse events. To keep the blood pressure down to the new 'normal' levels, people often had to take more than one type of drug and therefore had more chance of experiencing side effects.

The bottom line is that medicalisation in this case has led to overdiagnosis. Lowering cut-offs for disease and converting millions of people from normal to diseased provides no benefit and only increases the direct harms from the treatment and the indirect harms from labelling. And to make things worse, the focus on drug treatment of people with mild hypertension has taken the focus off other safer, cheaper and better treatments, such as weight loss and exercise.

Changing the definition of gestational diabetes

The changing cut-off for a diagnosis of type 2 diabetes provides another illustration of the unintended consequences of well-meaning attempts to treat more people and improve health. But while there's controversy about the definitions used for type 2 diabetes (the new diagnosis of 'pre-diabetes' is expected to result in 50 per cent of adults in China being diagnosed), it's gestational diabetes, diabetes diagnosed during pregnancy, that illustrates the problem best.

Gestational diabetes mellitus can occur during pregnancy in women who didn't have diabetes before the pregnancy, and presents risks for both the mother and the baby. It's usually diagnosed based on blood sugar levels and treated with drugs. It's also associated with more interventions, such as caesarean sections during delivery. In 2014, the cut-off blood sugar level for diagnosing gestational diabetes was lowered. This resulted in a more than doubling of the number of pregnant women diagnosed with gestational diabetes – women previously considered normal.

The benefits of changing the diagnostic criteria weren't made clear before changing them – it was done on the *presumption* of benefit. The US National Institutes for Health reviewed the scientific evidence and concluded there was no high-quality evidence that changing the criteria helps either mothers or babies. The costs of instituting the proposed changes were estimated to be billions of dollars. Furthermore, the overdiagnosis or labelling pregnant women with gestational diabetes has clear negative consequences, psychologically and physically (more interventions), and these have not been adequately considered or properly weighed against any potential benefits.

Pre-obesity

The WHO, using body mass index (BMI), a measure of obesity based on height and weight, classes those with a BMI of 25 to 30 as 'pre-obese'. By using that term, they are assuming that it's only a matter of time before everyone in that class will tip their BMI over the 30 mark into 'obese'. While this will certainly be true for some, it won't be so for everyone.

There's no doubt that obesity is associated with a wide range of diseases and that higher grades of obesity (a BMI over 35) are associated with many chronic health conditions and a higher risk of dying. But a review article examining the mortality risk of different categories of obesity found that being 'pre-obese' was associated with the lowest mortality, even lower than 'normal'. This finding has been challenged and may not represent cause and effect, but it's not indicating a major risk of dying from being pre-obese. While the label of 'pre-obesity' may act as a warning for some people, the balance of advantages and disadvantages with this label are still unclear.

Pre-fracture: osteopaenia

Osteopaenia (mild 'thinning' of the bones) is another condition that has no symptoms and is a normal ageing process. Osteopaenia is defined as a bone density lower than normal, but the definition gets tricky because it depends on what you call normal. Normal, in this case, is the bone density of a healthy young person, not people of a similar age (or gender or ethnicity). Osteopaenia is defined as being one 'standard deviation' below that of a normal young adult. As we have mentioned before, when the value falls to 2.5 standard deviations below normal, it's termed osteo*porosis*. Using these definitions, most post-menopausal women, and men of the same age for that matter, have or will soon have osteopaenia.

In 1992, when the WHO first proposed and defined osteopaenia (and created an alternative definition of osteoporosis based purely on a person's bone density rather than the traditional definition of having had a 'minimal trauma' fracture), it was never meant to be used as a diagnostic label or to have any treatment implications. As noted by Dr L Joseph Melton, an expert who participated in setting the criterion for osteopaenia, the cut-off was 'just meant to show a huge group who looked like they might be at risk'.

According to a 2003 *New York Times* article by Gina Kolata, 'Bone diagnosis gives new data but no answers', the new definition was meant to prompt governments to pay attention to the problem of bone loss. The article quoted another osteoporosis epidemiologist as saying, 'There is no basis, no biological, social, economic or treatment basis, no basis whatsoever, for using [the threshold]'. Unfortunately, that message seems to have been lost; more than half the population over the age of 50 have now been arbitrarily labelled with a disease, and many have been treated for it.

The diagnosis of osteopaenia, like osteoporosis, is centred on the idea that having thin bones predisposes people to fractures and that treating it prevents them. These fractures can occur nearly anywhere but most commonly in the wrist, foot, hip, spine and shoulder. The real disease – what we want to prevent – is fractures. Treating osteopaenia sounds like a good idea, but on closer inspection some things don't make sense.

Firstly, the treatment tends to rely on bone mineral density (BMD) measurements. But while a low BMD is a risk factor for having fractures, on its own it doesn't cause fractures. Falls are what most commonly cause fractures. As we saw in chapter 7, if people didn't fall, there would be significantly fewer fractures to worry about.

The correlation between bone density and fracture risk is not straightforward. This is because what we are measuring when we measure bone density is not the whole picture. The strength of a bone depends on lots of things, like the way the different cells and structures that make up bone are arranged and the size and the shape of the bone (which can change with age), not just how porous the bone is, which is what the test measures.

Secondly, the effectiveness of drug treatments in preventing fractures has only been proven in people who have already sustained a 'minimal trauma' fracture – defined as a fracture from a fall from at most standing height. People who sustain a minimal trauma fracture have a much higher chance of another fracture in the future, regardless of their bone density. The drug effectiveness, however, has not been proven for people who have been diagnosed with osteopaenia who haven't had any fractures. It should also be noted that the effective drugs used to prevent fractures *aren't* calcium and vitamin D, the ones commonly prescribed. Calcium, vitamin D and a combination of the two are generally not effective at reducing the chance of fracture. The drugs that do lower the chance of fracture, such as the bisphosphonates (e.g. alendronate [e.g. Fosamax], zolendronic acid [e.g. Aclasta] and the biologic drug denosumab [e.g. Prolia]) are much more expensive and are associated with more severe albeit uncommon adverse effects, such as avascular necrosis of the jaw (death of the bone tissue adjacent to the teeth due to an interruption of the blood supply) and spontaneous stress fractures of the femur (thigh bone).

Another problem is that although the effective drugs can increase the amount of bone a person has, therefore raising their BMD, they don't do it naturally. The most common of these drugs simply stops the process of the old bone being removed. But bones are constantly being remodelled and turned over on a microscopic level – that's how bones last so long and don't break easily. Bones commonly get microscopic stress fractures that are repaired before they become any bigger: old bone (including calcium) is always being removed and new bone laid down in its place – bone is a living tissue. That process is completely stopped when you take these drugs, and if you take them for long enough, stress fractures, causing pain or complete breaks, are *more* likely. These usually occur in the thigh bone, often in both thighs, and frequently require surgery. In fact, these fractures are harder to heal than the common types of fracture the drugs aim to prevent.

While these drugs can be effective even in people who have already had a fracture, for the most common type of drug, we have to treat 100 people for three years to prevent just one hip fracture, and most of the studies on these drugs have not included people older than 80, who make up the majority of those with hip fractures. These drugs probably prevent more fractures than they cause, especially now that we're more aware of the risks, but as you can see, it's not that simple.

These drugs are given to people with osteopaenia who are not at high risk of fracture, have not had a minimal trauma fracture and might have a very low risk of falling over. In these people the drugs are unlikely to be effective.

In 2008 there was a redefinition of who should get treatment. It was estimated that the changed criteria increased the proportion of white US women over 65 who should be treated with drugs from 21 to 72 per cent overnight, while also increasing the proportion or women over 75 to 93 per cent. This guideline, and many guidelines published since, rely on the BMD score and on the risk of a fracture in the future, rather than solely relying on having had a minimal trauma fracture or having osteoporosis. The usefulness of screening with BMD and with various fracture prediction tools has also been questioned, including in 2018 by the US Preventive Services Task Force, which makes recommendations about the effectiveness of specific preventive care services for people without obvious disease.

Our tendency to focus on treating one particular risk factor, or one particular set of measurable numbers, not only often leads to overtreatment and unnecessary harms but also has an 'opportunity cost'. In spending our time and money on one particular risk factor, we're not spending that time and money on other equally or more important factors. In the case of osteopaenia and osteoporosis, the focus is taken away from preventing falls.

Diagnosis creep

These shifting definitions of disease have been called 'diagnosis creep'. Studies have shown that the criteria for diagnosing diseases tend to always go in one direction – towards *widening* (not narrowing) the definition, diagnosing *more* (not fewer) people with disease. You have seen that there's often little evidence to support these recommendations and that the harms are often not well considered.

So why does it happen? While these changes are often aimed at improving health in more people, many of the new diagnoses can be treated with lifestyle and other modifications. Could it be a coincidence that these recommendations also help sell a lot more drugs? Is there a link between the drug companies and those making the recommendations? A review of recommendations to widen diagnostic guidelines for disease definitions showed that three-quarters of the experts on the panels had financial links to pharmaceutical companies, and half of them had links to at least seven companies each.

Socially constructed disease

So far, we have focused on overdiagnosis from the perspective of unnecessary but well-meaning medicalisation initiated by doctors to improve health. Overdiagnosis primarily occurs from *inside* medicine, although it can be influenced by cultural and societal norms. Medicalisation, on the other hand, is created by a specific set of cultural and social conditions and can be driven by forces both within and outside of medicine. Through our tendency to seek medical solutions to what are really social problems we often overlook solutions outside of medicine. This is illustrated by the medicalisation of obesity discussed in the previous chapter. By treating obesity within a medical framework, we tend to locate the source of the problem as lying within the individual (rather than within society), and we therefore direct solutions at the individual level (e.g. gastric surgery). We overlook the important non-medical factors that have contributed to the problem, where better solutions to the problem may lie.

Society's norms and values also influence our perception of health and what constitutes a medical problem. There are many historical and current examples of medicalising conditions that society believes to be 'wrong', 'deviant' or just 'different' and thereby justifying medical treatment. Medicine has also been used to justify and support racism and discrimination. For example, in 1851, the

Medical Association of Louisiana created a new diagnosis called 'drapetomania', a disease of the mind that made slaves run away. Presumably, that was the only explanation they could think of. The term remained in at least one medical dictionary until 1914. Whipping and the removal of both big toes were suggested remedies.

In the 20th century, it was not uncommon to forcibly sterilise people with genetic and sexual variations, HIV, low IQ and certain ethnicities, based on these characteristics being declared undesirable. These were carried out by doctors, but also often recommended by them. Forced sterilisation of ethnic minorities continues today. Peru instigated a 'family planning program' in 1996, a supposedly voluntary sterilisation of women under the guise of driving down poverty. Between 1996 and 2000, well over a quarter of a million women were reportedly sterilised, most of them from low-income Indigenous communities. According to Amnesty International, there's strong evidence that doctors were pressured to reach sterilisation quotas, and in most cases the women did not give their willing consent. Some doctors refused. In 2021, forced sterilisation (as well as abortion) is believed by international observers to be the explanation for the markedly falling birth rates among Uighur women in China.

Even masturbation in both men and women has been considered a disease. It has been blamed for many negative effects on the mind and body such as madness, idiocy, gout, epilepsy, back pain, headache, pimples and suicide. It has also been treated surgically in both men and women. It was only removed from the list of psychiatric diagnoses in 1968. Attempts to medicalise masturbation continue today, based on questionable evidence.

We've touched on many examples of medicalising normal. Some have been well intentioned but misguided, some have been influenced by the societal norms of the time, while others have had far less noble motives. In painting medical treatment as the answer to many of life's problems, normal predicaments and annoyances of life are converted into medical conditions that need treating. Almost any departure from average can be medicalised, from sexual performance or pleasure to bowel habits, pain, sadness, or appearance (e.g. baldness).

It's worth reflecting on the harms that have arisen from the application of medicalised labels over the years given that few of the people to whom they were applied had any complaints in the first place. Current examples arise when someone *other* than the 'affected' person complains. Parents often worry about their children and may pursue diagnosis of an eating disorder for minor changes in eating behaviour. A diagnosis can be easy to make when the definitions are as unhelpful as that for binge eating disorder, defined as eating, in a two-hour period, an amount of food that's definitely more than most people would eat in a similar period under similar circumstances.

* * *

The pledge of the Hippocratic Oath discussed in this chapter reminds doctors that they have responsibility not only to those who are infirm, but also to those who are 'sound of mind and body'. Doctors are given a powerful place in society and are in a position to influence society as a whole. They can use this influence to avoid medicalising healthy people. In medicalising normal, labelling people unnecessarily, and prescribing treatments that enrich themselves and harm patients, they are betraying their pledge to society.

10

Healing

Hippocratic Oath: If I do not violate this oath, may I enjoy life and art, respected while I live and remembered with affection thereafter. May I always act so as to preserve the finest traditions of my calling and may I long experience the joy of healing those who seek my help.

'Wherever the art of medicine is loved,
there is also a love of humanity'
– attributed to Hippocrates

We love our roles as doctors. We regularly experience the joy of healing – for example, by watching a fracture heal in good alignment after surgical fixation, or seeing a case of severe inflammatory arthritis resolve with modern drugs – and we want to preserve the trust we enjoy. We also want to make it clear that we believe that most, if not all doctors, are trying to help their patients, not harm them.

Although we've given many examples of the ways doctors are failing to live up to the Hippocratic Oath, we haven't set out to deliberately erode trust in doctors. Rather, our aim has been to bring knowledge of the problems with modern medicine to a wider audience in the hope that by understanding the problems, we can focus on what needs to change. We would like many more doctors (and patients) to experience that 'joy of healing' that comes from a more *science-informed* understanding of the *true* benefits of medicine and its *true* harms.

The problems with modern medicine have many potential solutions. There are things patients can do and things doctors need to do. There are also things society and the system – by which we mean governments, funders, industry, universities and researchers – need to do.

What can patients do?

Patients need to demand that their voices be heard and their views considered, and they need to be involved as actively as they can. The focus should be on patient-relevant needs and outcomes in all aspects of health care, from individual decision-making to decisions about national policy.

Be informed and inform others

Before they can be involved, patients, carers and the public need to be informed. Of course, it's hard to be informed if you don't know there's a problem, which is why we wrote this book.

As we've seen, most patients subscribe to the belief that more care (tests and treatments) leads to better health. Like their doctors, they generally overestimate the benefits of a test or treatment and underestimate the harms. In fact, many people are unaware that simply doing a test can lead to harm. While some of this preference for 'more' medicine is understandably driven by fear and a desire for the avoidance of anticipated regret – both strong motivators for choosing tests or treatments over doing nothing – we hope this book moderates these beliefs.

Patients also need to ensure their doctors are adequately informed about *them*. At an individual doctor–patient level they must make their concerns and wishes clear and ensure that their doctors acknowledge and consider them. On a broader level, some countries now have national health records to which patients can contribute. One example is My Health Record (<myhealthrecord. gov.au>) in Australia. This system contains information about medical conditions, past and current treatments, test results, allergies and treatment preferences, including advanced care directives written by patients, in which they can state their preferences for future treatment in certain situations. All this information is available to treating doctors. These systems can help minimise wasteful and erroneous treatment.

Patients should *demand* and expect to *receive* full and accurate information on the potential benefits *and* harms of any test or treatment that a doctor or someone else recommends. For complex or difficult decisions, they could ask their doctor for a decision aid to help them make test or treatment choices, or they could search for these themselves. Patients should never be afraid to ask for a second opinion. Many patients consider a second opinion to be an insult to their doctor, but doctors are usually grateful for second opinions and can become more comfortable with their own decision-making when it agrees with recommendations from a colleague, or when they're forced to reconsider or defend their decision if a colleague disagrees. We don't know any doctors who think second opinions are a bad idea.

As well as being fully informed, patients have a right to be actively involved in decision-making about their health together with their doctor. Patients should realise that they have the autonomy to make decisions for themselves and they should exercise that right.

Many questions might be helpful for a patient to ask a doctor (see the reference list for this chapter). The most important one when considering a test or treatment is: what is the evidence that this test or treatment will be better for my health compared to not doing it or using other, safer treatments? This critical question often goes unasked by the patient and the doctor, but it lies at the heart of science. To phrase it another way, what's the balance of benefits and harms for this proposed test or treatment compared to the alternatives, including doing nothing?

Choosing Wisely Australia, one of many national voices for reducing unnecessary tests and treatments in health care, recommends five simple questions that separate out the different parts of this critical question:

1 Do I really need this test, treatment or procedure?
   (i.e. What are the possible benefits?)
2 What are the risks? (i.e. What are the possible harms?)
3 Are there simpler, safer options?
4 What happens if I don't do anything?
5 What are the costs?

Noting that many patients may be uncomfortable asking questions, Choosing Wisely Australian spokesperson Robyn Lindner recommends that the focus be on promoting conversations between patients and their doctors or other healthcare providers.

We don't want to force people to ask questions. Clinicians need to be aware that they must provide the space and support for these conversations, knowing that their patients may not be comfortable asking the questions themselves.

Improve your own knowledge

Many people struggle with finding and assessing medical evidence, which is why education in the principles of science, or 'science literacy', is so important. An understanding of science is needed to appreciate how evidence is generated and appraised and to know what high-quality, trustworthy evidence looks like.

A lack of scientific understanding makes people vulnerable to misinformation. And when this occurs at a global level it's a major threat to public health. Misinformation about COVID-19 is rife, for example. A recent study using large national surveys in the United States, United Kingdom, Ireland, Spain and Mexico found that higher trust in scientists and higher numeracy skills were associated with lower susceptibility to coronavirus-related misinformation. There was also a clear link between susceptibility to misinformation and both vaccine hesitancy and a reduced likelihood of complying with health guidance measures.

Science literacy can be improved by improving education in general, but knowledge of science can be easily gained on the internet: everything from university courses to blogs and chat rooms can help. Wikipedia is a good source of evidence-based information: it is regularly updated, and custodians of the information ensure that, as much as possible, it is free from bias.

Science is like a toolkit, an instruction set that helps us reduce error (get the 'least wrong' answer) when we try to create new knowledge. Like any tool, it must be used properly, and the more we use it, the more proficient we become. Perhaps the most important advice we can give to anyone who wishes to be more scientific is to start by questioning things. Don't take anything as proven or granted. And don't just question things you already don't believe – that's too easy; start questioning the things you *do* believe. Questioning doesn't mean 'not believing'. Questioning means applying the scientific tools of critical thinking and reasoning to the things you believe.

As well as science literacy, our ability to be actively involved in decisions about our health is dependent on our 'health literacy'. This is our motivation and ability to access, understand and use health information in order to make the best decisions for our health. Health literacy dictates the extent to which we can determine what's true and useful, how we understand probability and risk, and how we manage interactions and communication with health professionals.

In our work surveying hundreds of people, we have found that most people struggle with the ability to access the *right* information and *use* it correctly – to understand it, appraise it and apply it. This even applies to those with high levels of education. Uniformly, irrespective of background, patients report difficulty in comparing health information from different sources and determining whether the information is credible and accurate. This makes them highly susceptible to misleading information on health websites and direct-to-consumer advertising about tests and treatments that promise to improve quality of life and/or extend life expectancy.

Most people also have little understanding of the role of bias or commercial interests in the promotion of unnecessary care. Irrespective of where the information comes from, people should consider its scientific strength; this is where critical appraisal skills help. While much of the information on the internet is unreliable and misleading, there's also plenty of accurate high-quality information if you know where to look. A broad collection of decision aids is available, for example, at <decisionaid.ohri.ca/AZlist.html>.

The *types* of evidence provided on a topic can also give you an idea about the scientific quality of the information. Be wary of information about tests and treatments that includes *no* mention of the evidence or, for that matter, of the potential *harms*. Tests and treatments usually have both benefits and harms, treatment comparisons should be fair, as in comparing like with like, and single studies can be misleading.

Some patient information resources ensure a high standard of quality, making the job of the patients a little easier. Personal opinions, if unsupported by evidence, may be unreliable. Good summaries of medical research can be found in the form of systematic reviews, but even then, not all systematic reviews are trustworthy.

Systematic reviews and the Cochrane Library

Many of the most trustworthy systematic reviews of medical studies are published in the Cochrane Library (<www.cochranelibrary. com>). The Cochrane Collaboration is an international organisation that's registered as a charity in the United Kingdom. It was established in 1993 and has more than 80000 contributors worldwide, mostly volunteers, based across 120 countries. It's not-for-profit and accepts no commercial funding. There are more than 50 review groups, each based around a field of medicine. We can vouch for the high quality of the Cochrane Library because of our many years of involvement. Rachelle has been the coordinating editor for Cochrane Musculoskeletal since 2005, and she herself has written more than a hundred Cochrane reviews.

Although the Cochrane Library is subscription-based, a program set up by the WHO provides free or low-cost access for most low- and middle-income countries. In many other parts of the world, including Australia, the library is freely available to all residents, thanks to governments paying the licence fee. Residents of all countries have free access to the summaries that accompany each Cochrane review, and lay summaries are provided. During the COVID pandemic, Cochrane has made its library temporarily available for everyone in every country of the world.

Be more involved

Patients can also be involved in decision-making at a higher level than just their own care, such as through government committees that involve patients or that put their findings out for public comment. Patients can join health consumer groups, but they should be aware of any conflicts that may arise from the financing of these groups by industry. It has been shown that most consumer groups that receive industry support don't acknowledge this.

Patients can also be a powerful lobbying force for political change, which can be used to promote effective care and reduce harmful care. They can also be a voice for system change through the ballot box. Some of the biggest political debates in the United States, over universal health care, immigration, gun control and abortion, all have enormous public health implications. There are many other important public debates with health implications, such as those concerning the pricing, labelling and advertising of food, tobacco and alcohol; and environmental regulations.

Research is traditionally the domain of academics, but it's now seen as beneficial for patients to be involved in research, not just as participants but as investigators. Most local research ethics committees will also have layperson members, which gives these members a good grasp of clinical science and current research. It's becoming more common for patients to be on research teams as investigators in their own right. This gives them a better understanding of the science involved in generating research, but importantly, as we discussed in chapter 7, can also make the research more relevant to future patients. In fact, altruism (a concern for others) has been shown to be one of the main reasons why people join research projects. Through involving patients and the public in the process, research will become more applicable to the general community, more rapidly taken up into practice, less wasteful, and ask the right scientific questions.

The Cochrane Collaboration involves patients in all aspects of its work. Of particular interest might be Cochrane Crowd (<crowd.cochrane.org/index.html>). In fact, anyone can become a 'Cochrane citizen scientist'. To date, almost 10 000 volunteers from 189 countries have done so. Volunteers help categorise and summarise healthcare evidence and can volunteer for a few minutes of their day or longer. Doctors can also become Cochrane citizen scientists. No experience is necessary; you learn on the job and get to contribute to medicine at the same time.

What can doctors do?

At an individual level, doctors can improve the quality of the doctor–patient interaction by reflecting on the content and the process of their communication with patients.

Inform patients

By providing information that patients can understand and by making use of written and visual information available in the office or online, doctors can enhance patient understanding and increase their satisfaction with decision-making.

In traditional medical systems, doctors were the authoritative figures who instructed patients about what care they should receive and when, and patients played a passive role. Since the 1970s and 1980s, there has been a shift towards both the patient and physician contributing to a shared medical decision-making process. This process still recognises the healthcare provider as an expert, but much more emphasis is placed on patients being best placed to understand their needs and which of the alternative care options might best align with their unique cultural and personal beliefs and their personal circumstances. While not everyone has embraced the concept of medical shared decision-making, a review of 115 studies published in 2012 found that patient acceptance of this approach has increased over time.

According to a Cochrane systematic review that included 105 studies, patients who use decision aids (interventions that make the shared decision-making much more explicit) have more accurate perceptions of benefits and risks and feel more confident in their health choices. Furthermore, there are no harmful effects on either health outcomes or satisfaction with care.

Be effective knowledge communicators

Doctors are the most frequently relied upon and trusted source of information for their patients. To be effective knowledge translators for patients – that is, to *communicate* effectively – they must understand their patient's health literacy. Failure to do so likely results in healthcare disparities.

Studies comparing doctors' best guesses about their patients' health literacy with the results from tools that directly measure it have found that the guesstimate is often way off the mark. Doctors tend to underestimate health literacy among minority groups. In general, however, predictors of suboptimal health literacy include lower education level, having been born overseas and/ or not speaking the language of their country of residence, social isolation, and the lack of an established relationship with at least one health professional. Patients with multiple health problems or comorbidities, a history of anxiety and depression, and/or poorer health behaviours, are also more likely to have suboptimal levels of health literacy.

Most doctors incorrectly believe that their patients have understood and will retain detailed information provided in a consultation, but as much as 80 per cent of the information won't be retained and up to half of what is retained will be remembered incorrectly. People with low health literacy are the population most at risk, but so are people who are anxious and those receiving bad news. Doctors suggesting that patients bring a 'second pair of ears' to the consultation can be helpful. Providing information in the form of decision aids, and the inclusion of explicit information on overdiagnosis can lead to a greater likelihood of patients making informed choices.

Doctors can improve accurate understanding of their message by using language the patient understands; avoiding technical, medical terms unless they are fully explained; and avoiding the use of rhetoric to sway patient decision-making. Checking to confirm that patients have understood the information as intended is also crucial.

Use of methods such as 'teach back' (also called 'show me') has been proven to improve doctor–patient communication, including retention of information by the patient. 'Teach back' is an interview approach that involves asking the patient to repeat the information a clinician has provided in their own words. This helps ensure that the clinician has provided information that can be understood. These strategies are particularly important in caring for people with poor health literacy. They're also useful for ensuring that what the doctor has heard from the patient is also understood as intended. Being fully informed works *both ways*, and has positive benefits for both the patient and the doctor.

Increasing empathy and compassion in the delivery of health care can also be successfully taught, so consideration should be given to obtaining these skills and setting up a practice that allows their delivery, for example by having longer consultation times.

Be science-based

Professor Sir John Tooke, a prominent English doctor best known for leading the Modernising Medical Careers inquiry, wrote, 'The doctor's role as diagnostician and the handler of clinical uncertainty and ambiguity requires a profound educational base in science and evidence-based practice as well as research awareness'.

Doctors too need to be sceptical. A better understanding of science will allow doctors to recognise errors that lie in personal observations and the observations of others due to confirmation bias, and how that error can be minimised by using scientific methods, including experimentation and comparative analysis. Properly appraising research is difficult and not always well taught in medical training, but it's an essential skill. It doesn't come naturally, but it can be learned and it must be practised. Many universities offer doctors face-to-face and online courses of varying length in clinical epidemiology. These courses include scientific methods for clinical research and critical appraisal of the medical literature. Courses in public health also include these relevant topics.

Scientific enquiry starts with a question; doctors must question current practice and determine if their practice is sufficiently supported by scientific evidence. They should start by asking whether *any* tests or treatments are warranted at this moment, before asking 'What is the evidence for this test or treatment compared to an alternative?'

Doctors also need to be able to find evidence when it exists. This requires them to be skilled in searching the scientific literature for the most valid and relevant specific studies related to their practice. Many practice guidelines and summaries are available, including systematic reviews, but doctors also need the appraisal skills to determine whether or not these are trustworthy.

In recognising that public health measures have a greater impact on health than much of modern medicine, it's also timely for doctors to consider the bigger questions, such as whether they should be spending less time investing their energy in 'fighting disease' and more time 'promoting health'. This requires an understanding of the difference between being illness-focused and being health-focused, and broadening the definition of health to encompass more than just the absence of a disease or control of a symptom.

Be involved in research

Doctors also have a responsibility to generate the evidence that underpins their practice. Too many doctors see research as something separate from the practice of medicine, but clinical practice and clinical research are the same thing. They are scientific endeavours aimed at finding and implementing the best treatments for people. In the United Kingdom for example, it's considered a doctor's duty to be involved in research and it's enshrined in the principles of the NHS.

Many benefits come from participating in clinical research. From the doctor's perspective it provides access to a network of other clinicians and researchers involved in research, which means they can benchmark their practice against others, while also providing an avenue to discuss difficult clinical problems. There are also benefits for patients. Not only may they be able to access promising new treatments earlier, but they have better outcomes. One study found that patients admitted to research-active UK hospitals for acute conditions had lower rates of dying compared with those in hospitals that weren't research-active.

To practise evidence-based medicine is to practise science-based medicine. The skills required to appraise scientific research are the same skills required to perform scientific research. Being actively involved in research not only facilitates the production of evidence, but increases awareness of evidence and knowledge of scientific methods, therefore increasing critical appraisal skills.

Reduce wasteful research

The scientific *quality* of research also needs to be improved and wasteful research reduced. Many doctors participate in research of low quality or that isn't relevant to clinical practice, or they conduct good research that's never published and therefore remains hidden from view. These factors contribute to research waste, where energy is expended in producing research unlikely to benefit anybody. If patients have been involved then this is also unethical.

Unfortunately, many doctors have insufficient understanding of these factors, including the elements that contribute to research quality, which is why science literacy is crucial for all doctors. Common errors include asking unimportant questions that are unlikely to benefit health; not establishing the need for the research in the first place by performing a systematic review, which might find the question has already been answered; not establishing the feasibility of the research before starting; and having insufficient people in the study to be able to draw definitive, or at least meaningful results.

By mid-2021, there were well over 9000 ongoing or completed COVID-19 studies, according to the WHO's International Clinical Trials Registry Platform. Despite the plethora of research related to COVID-19, much of it is opportunistic and not relevant to improving patient care.

Research should address important health problems, use the highest quality methods and be focused on important patient-relevant outcomes. It should also be implementable, meaning that if appropriate, the results can easily be introduced into clinical practice and cause real change. Doctors, as well as patients, can make valuable contributions to research projects to make them more clinically relevant. They can also contribute to disseminating the results and increasing their uptake into practice.

Justify their elevated position

Doctors have high status and considerable power in society. This position comes with a responsibility to society that they can fulfil by properly managing the resources under their control. They should only introduce new diagnoses and treatments once there's adequate evidence of a clear benefit, with full consideration of known and possibly unintended harms. They should be patient-centred rather than practise defensive medicine. Treating the 'worried well' or those without suspicious symptoms with more tests and diagnoses, rather than identifying and treating their underlying anxiety, is counterproductive and likely to be harmful.

Doctors should also be aware of potential and actual conflicts of interest and where possible, remove them. Such conflicts have been shown to negatively influence practice, and doctors need to understand that simply *declaring* conflicts of interest does not remove or negate them.

Doctors' status in society is such that they are trusted with self-regulation, but to truly deserve this position, doctors need to hold themselves to a higher standard. They need to practise humility and be aware of and address their own deficiencies. Financial conflicts, personal biases, poor communication, and lack of scientific rigour all need to be addressed.

Support the Choosing Wisely campaign

The Choosing Wisely campaign is noteworthy because it is directed specifically at improving value in care and was started by *doctors*. One of its foundational principles is that sometimes the most effective treatment a physician can offer is sage advice, rather than doing a test, prescribing a medicine or performing an operation.

The campaign was established in response to a 2010 perspective piece in the *New England Journal of Medicine* by Dr Howard Brody, a US ethicist and family doctor. In 'Medicine's ethical responsibility for health care reform – the top five list', Dr Brody wrote that it was the ethical duty of physicians to take the lead in identifying wasteful healthcare practices. He proposed that each medical specialty society identify five tests and treatments that were overused in their specialties and provided no meaningful benefit for patients. The first list of its kind was published the following year by three US primary care specialties, family medicine, internal medicine and paediatrics.

The American Board of Internal Medicine Foundation launched the Choosing Wisely campaign in 2012. Recognising that up to 30 per cent of health care is wasteful, the initiative promotes doctor–patient conversations that will help patients avoid unnecessary medical tests and treatments and choose care that's supported by evidence, free from harm and truly necessary. Wendy Levinson, Professor of Medicine at the University of Toronto and chair of Choosing Wisely Canada, has said, 'Choosing Wisely goes back to the core essence of being a clinician – having conversations with your patients'.

The underlying framework of the Choosing Wisely campaign is a new physician charter, 'Medical professionalism in the new millennium: a physician charter'. While the Hippocratic Oath focuses on care for the individual, this new charter emphasises that doctors have responsibilities *beyond* the individual patient. This includes promotion of the just distribution of finite resources, managing conflicts of interest and improving quality of care. These principles recognise and address the escalating costs of health care and the large waste due to overtreatment, which deprives the undertreated of necessary care. It also adds a commitment to transparency and shared decision-making. We have included these concepts in our discussions throughout the book.

More than 20 countries, including Australia, now have their own Choosing Wisely campaigns. There are now well over a thousand recommendations against wasteful tests and procedures. Sharing this information among peers and patients is vital for reducing these ingrained practices in health care. There has also been much emphasis on partnering with consumer organisations to produce easy-to-read brochures and patient stories and other materials for the general public.

Reduce medicine's environmental impact

Individual doctors and professional societies can also play a crucial role in minimising the negative impact their care has on the environment. Many doctors are already leading by example in many ways. In Australia, Doctors for the Environment Australia (DEA;

<www.dea.org.au>) and the Climate and Health Alliance (CAHA; <www.caha.org.au>) are committed to educating, informing and influencing governments, industry, the public and colleagues of the need to address climate change. Reducing the environmental impact of too much medical care is intrinsic to this goal. Both the DEA and the Australian Medical Association (AMA) have called on the federal government to establish a Sustainable Development Unit to develop and implement a national carbon reduction plan to reduce our high-carbon healthcare system. This could be based on the United Kingdom's Unit, which reduced carbon emissions by 11 per cent from 2008 to 2018, despite activity increasing by 18 per cent. It has also saved at least £90 million annually. Doctors and other frontline clinicians and staff were integral to the plan, which covered a wide range of issues from energy and carbon management to food procurement, travel plans and waste management. Reducing overprescribing and overtreatment was integral to the plan.

What can medical professional societies do?

Medicine is largely self-regulated when it comes to education and standards, and these tasks are often left to the specialist medical societies, colleges, academies and associations, which themselves decide who can be a member, based on education and practice standards. There are fundamental problems with self-regulation, such as the conflict between a society serving its members and serving society as a whole.

Unfortunately, the current system of self-regulation lacks teeth and depth when it comes to these groups enforcing their own standards. No society ever kicked out a doctor for being a bad scientist, but that doesn't mean that they can't start demanding and enforcing some standards. In one instance, Rachelle received a much delayed apology from a professional society for the behaviour of a doctor while he was acting on behalf of the society. The letter stated that the offender had met with the Professional Conduct and Standards Committee and had been made aware that his behaviour had been unprofessional and unfitting for a representative of the society. The doctor had been required to complete an 'operating with respect' education course and was a signatory on an apology letter from the society, but he continues in representative roles. Unfortunately, the policing of scientific standards in clinical practice is even less rigorous.

Requirements for specialist accreditation and practice are often based on qualifications, knowledge in examinations and practice reviews. This is an ideal mechanism to start ensuring adequacy of scientific knowledge (such as knowledge of research methods and skills in critical appraisal). Professional societies should broaden their requirements beyond specialty-based skills and knowledge to include mandatory science literacy.

Professional societies can also influence their members' practice with the practice guidelines and recommendations many commonly produce. They often also provide evidence-based patient education information and nominate expert members to other (for example, government) committees charged with developing health policy.

What can society and the system do?

While individual changes by both patients and doctors can make a significant impact, systemic change is also of vital importance.

Media

To ensure that medicine is reported more reliably in the media we require better science literacy among journalists. Journalists may also benefit from a closer relationship with researchers and should avoid using commentators without the appropriate, unbiased expertise. The current competitive media environment and its underlying business model make it difficult to realise this goal. Income depends on circulation and click-throughs, which reward sensationalism over responsible scientific reporting. There's also a problem with the longstanding practice of not wanting to appear biased by always including an opposing view, even when that view is wrong.

Governments

Governments have enormous power to influence health through various avenues, many of which are common to other groups, depending on the jurisdiction. The government role in each of these will vary between and within countries. Governments are probably best placed to address the problem of the business model under which medicine is conducted, whereby profits (and therefore costs and throughput) are maximised, perverse incentives prevail and doctors create demand rather than satisfy it.

Healthcare funding

Healthcare funders tend to behave *reactively* – funding health based on the demand from the system, demand that largely arises from doctors. The health dollar could be better spent by analysing the value received for the money that is spent. Disinvesting in low-value care and investing the savings in high-value care is a current focus for many health funders. To do this effectively, value must be adequately measured. This is difficult because of limited data availability, variable data quality and the fact that much of the routinely collected data is based on processes – that is, costs, length of stay, and numbers of tests and procedures performed – rather than health-based outcomes such as patient-reported health and the appropriateness of tests and treatments.

Funders do have the capacity to determine value in health

care. They have the capacity to generate evidence in this area and make better use of the massive data available to them. By encouraging the use of standardised electronic data capture, making data access easier, making data systems more compatible and enabling linkage between systems, they can leverage routinely collected data to generate information on the value of health interventions. Kaiser Permanente in the United States, for example, has invested billions of dollars in information technology to track the health and care of its members. Being a closed, integrated network of doctors, hospitals, diagnostic services and pharmacies allows Kaiser to obtain a complete picture. Using these data has allowed the company to focus on the best-value treatments and prevention based on patient-important health outcomes. And it has been able to provide relatively low-cost care with better health outcomes than other, less integrated health insurance systems.

Many funding bodies throughout the world have been tasked with determining the 'value' or cost-effectiveness or relative effectiveness of medical interventions. Because of the complexity of the work involved, these groups can often evaluate only a limited number of interventions. These groups often make their work publicly available; see, for example, Cochrane Health Technology Assessments (<cochranelibrary-wiley.com/o/cochrane/cochrane_clhta_articles_fs.html>), the UK National Institute for Health and Care Excellence (NICE) (<www.nice.org.uk>), the US Preventive Services Task Force (<www.uspreventiveservicestaskforce.org>) and Health Evidence (<healthevidence.org>).

Healthcare funders should strengthen evidence requirements *before* agreeing to fund or subsidise new tests and treatments. Healthcare funders have found that lack of effectiveness *alone* is not sufficient to withdraw treatments that they subsidise when it goes against the ingrained current beliefs of the doctors. Apart from the pushback from doctors, patients assume that coverage means the treatments must be effective.

At a minimum, funders should require at least two high-quality randomised controlled trials and, wherever feasible, at least one of these should include a placebo control. In the absence of high-quality evidence, they could consider sponsoring trials themselves and providing coverage for the new treatment only if the patient is participating in a study testing whether it works. Early engagement with patients, clinicians and professional societies to build support for the trial and its design would build science literacy as well.

Some countries have recently reviewed government subsidisation of tests and procedures, targeting areas of low-value care. A review of Medicare's Medical Benefits Schedule in Australia is in the process of removing support for some procedures. Similar UK reviews have restricted access to 18 treatments declared low value (including tonsillectomy for sore throats, hysterectomy for heavy menstrual bleeding, knee arthroscopy for osteoarthritis, surgery for bone spurs in the shoulder and steroid injections in the spine), which will save £200 million per year. More attention could be given to ways of rewarding evidence-based practice by developing innovative payment initiatives. Further research into geographic variation in clinical practice can also identify and target areas of overuse or underuse.

And finally, if we're to reduce the harms from medicine, we need to measure them better. Most of the research into medical harms so far has come from pulling hospital files and reading through them. Now that records are electronic, we should be able to automatically detect harms: falls, pressure ulcers, medication reactions, infections, clots and even previously hard to measure outcomes such as patient dissatisfaction. Using large datasets of routinely collected data, governments and regulators can start to measure unnecessary care and its harms more accurately.

Research funding

Funders of health research are in a position to reduce research waste, and to fund projects that address major health problems and are most likely to result in health improvements. The Netherlands government has introduced a system for reimbursing new or unproven treatments by requiring that an evaluation be undertaken (which the government also funds). Stakeholders, including patients and doctors, agree at the outset on the evidence that would be required, including the types of patients that should be treated and the outcomes that should be assessed. This recently resulted in the initial subsidisation and later removal of a specific technique, radiofrequency denervation, to address back pain, after two trials found it was no better than placebo. One per cent of the UK NHS budget is devoted to providing support for research within the NHS. This has been very successful in improving the uptake of research findings into practice.

As mentioned for individual researchers, funders should ensure they avoid research waste by funding research that's feasible, addresses an important issue, is of high quality and can be implemented. They should also ensure that the results of the research they fund are widely available. They should insist on publication of all findings, preferably in an open-access rather than pay-per-view format.

Research funders and universities should also consider what they can do to protect and support the researchers they fund. Individual researchers need better protection against vested interests, and a process for how this can be enacted. Possible strategies could include a hotline for advice and support. Researchers need to know they're supported, and also their rights and avenues for redress.

Several junior researchers who have been intimidated for their research declined our invitation to tell their stories in this book. They feared it would jeopardise their careers and ability to attract research funding. With increasing acceptance of the need to evaluate the value of medical practice in high-quality studies, it's likely that more researchers will come under fire from those who have a vested interest in the results. This may reduce the pool of people willing to pursue a clinical research career.

Regulation

The regulatory environment for research needs overhauling. The necessary ethical and governance hurdles required for research into the effectiveness of new cancer drugs, for example, are also applied to simple studies comparing two commonly used treatments. This creates unnecessary obstacles for those who wish to perform simple research comparing the effectiveness of common, well-known and safe treatments for their relative effectiveness. We would argue that where there's variation in the way certain conditions are managed, it's unethical to continue treating people differently without doing a structured study that properly compares the results of the different approaches.

Interestingly, if a doctor developed a new type of surgery (say, a new way of doing a hip replacement), they could start doing it without needing ethics committee approval. But if that same surgeon wanted to find out if it was any good, by contacting patients at a later date and, say, comparing them to patients that they had treated with the old type of surgery, they would come up against considerable regulatory hurdles. For a start, they would require full ethics committee approval to contact their own patients for such a purpose. The current system makes it very difficult to do the research, and very easy to simply continue treating people differently, never knowing which treatment is best. Changes in this area would significantly reduce the burden on researchers and remove an important obstruction to conducting timely, low-risk research.

Greater consideration should be given to influencing health using methods outside the direct, individual delivery of health interventions or research. Health can be improved, and health costs reduced, through prevention strategies aimed at major determinants of health, such as obesity, physical exercise and drug use, including tobacco and alcohol.

Policies aimed at improving the public's knowledge can have a strong positive impact on the health of society. It's estimated that about half of US adults have difficulty understanding and acting on health information, a problem strongly related to literacy and numeracy in general. Due to this and many other factors, there's a strong correlation between a person's level of education and their health. People with higher levels of education have a better understanding of the things that influence their health, such as diet, exercise and smoking, and they interact with health systems with much less difficulty. Health literacy and health in general are both closely related to education status.

Consideration should also be given to medical malpractice laws. In New Zealand, Denmark and Sweden, for example, a compensation system has replaced the use of the courts and the associated high insurance premiums for medical malpractice. These systems are not associated with higher-than-average medical harms, and defensive medicine is less common in these environments. The running costs for a medical practice are also lower, removing another incentive to overtreat. As discussed in chapter 4, the control of doctors through malpractice law fails to address the problems discussed in this book.

External regulation of doctors, for example by government licensing, is a better system to control doctors, as it covers all doctors and is arguably more open to change than the legal system. It can also address the gap in regulation that has come from allowing doctors to self-regulate.

The track record of external regulation has shown that this avenue is usually reserved for the 'bad apples' (often those who make fraudulent and implausibly excessive claims for rendered services), not the average doctor who's just doing what everyone else is doing. Getting regulators to police medicalisation might be a big stretch, but there are some things large regulators can do.

Firstly, they can oversee the professional societies and set standards for their oversight of their members. They can also promote professionalism and responsibility at the time of licensing. In many countries, the government also oversees medical training, another opportunity to promote science-based practice and raise awareness of the extent and causes of medical harm.

The Australian Department of Health has recently employed the use of audit and feedback letters to curb overtesting and overtreatment. The intent of this approach is to invite doctors identified as being 'high prescribers' to *reflect* upon their practice relative to their peers, as a quality-improvement exercise. A Cochrane review summarising the effectiveness of audit and feedback based on 140 studies indicates that, on average, this can increase the desired practice by about 4 per cent (a sizeable amount at a population level).

Topics have included antibiotic prescribing for the common cold, opioid prescriptions and imaging for musculoskeletal conditions. These letters compare the number of tests or prescriptions of the doctor to their peers in a similar geographic region and also provide evidence-based recommendations and resources to help them change their practice if appropriate. Follow-up letters show how their practices may have changed over time.

There have been some critics of this approach. For a start, it invokes fear among those who receive a letter. Feedback is also more effective when delivered by a trusted colleague or supervisor (not the Chief Medical Officer of Australia). As well, the method for identifying high prescribers is very crude, and cannot distinguish appropriate from inappropriate high use according to the needs of the patients the doctor serves. Nevertheless, the results have been encouraging and the accumulating experience and more recent high-quality evaluations of the audit and feedback letters (performed in collaboration with the Wiser Healthcare collaboration), will inform improvements to the program.

Hospitals and other healthcare organisations

Many of the solutions that apply to doctors, health funders and regulators also apply to hospitals and other healthcare organisations. Firstly, there appears to be a link between research engagement and healthcare performance. As noted earlier, research-active trusts in the United Kingdom provide better care and have lower mortality for acute hospital admissions compared to centres that aren't research-active. Research-active trusts with the highest level of research funding also have far lower mortality rates than those with less research funding. They're also more likely to provide care that better aligns with practice guidelines, and hospitals with research networks will implement evidence into practice faster and more easily. It has been suggested that research-active hospitals accumulate greater knowledge, develop better infrastructure, and can bring in resources that can improve clinical care more broadly. Encouraging research networks in hospitals is win-win.

To provide optimal care, healthcare organisations must, like doctors, understand the needs and preferences of their patients. Information about the health literacy of their patients can offer hospitals and other healthcare organisations insights into the challenges people experience when trying to access and engage with their services. This may help them identify ways to enhance the engagement of patients in their health and health care, thus improving health outcomes.

One worthwhile approach, after determining patient health literacy, is for the hospital or healthcare organisation to involve their staff in generating and testing potential interventions to meet the specific needs of their patients. In one of our studies, involving workshops with the health professionals who actually care for patients in nine different healthcare organisations, between 21 and 78 intervention ideas per organisation were generated to address the specific health literacy needs of their patients.

These ideas involved developing clinician skills and resources for health literacy; engaging community volunteers to disseminate health messages; directly improving consumer health literacy, for example by offering classes in searching for good medical information on the internet; and redesigning existing services. Each organisation then implemented and progressively refined one intervention idea, and was able to demonstrate meaningful health-service improvements.

To adopt this approach, health literacy questions could be included in the standard hospital pre-admission form and integrated into pathway planning. Relevant staff could be required to complete mandatory health literacy training, and dedicated staff, or even trained volunteer advocates, could be employed to help people identified as having specific health literacy needs.

Hospitals can also optimise evidence-based practice through educational, process and regulatory strategies, and monitor practice variation under their roof. Before investing in new technology for tests or treatments, hospitals should consider the comparative effectiveness and safety of these advances in comparison to the present technologies, whether they are likely to have any unintended harmful consequences, and whether the finances might be better spent elsewhere. The focus here should be on improving health rather than introducing new tests and treatments to improve reputation or profit.

Audit and feedback strategies to reduce low-value care could be set up in hospitals. Some states in Australia are already investing in and investigating this approach through data platforms and dashboards. These can provide data to the clinicians in real time to improve patient care.

Hospitals also have a major role in ensuring the environmental sustainability of health care. Even when medical care is beneficial to the person receiving it, it may cause unintended health harms on others. Some Australian states have already recognised the need to reduce greenhouse gas emissions caused by the health system and produced strategy plans.

Industry

The profit motive in industry promotes higher costs and higher consumption of health care over the optimisation of health. This has led to ineffective and harmful treatments and low-value care.

While industry plays an important role in the development of new treatments and the efficient production of drugs and devices, industry needs to remain separate from the regulatory environment that controls the *use* of these drugs and devices. In some countries, such as the United States, the drug regulator (the FDA) is mostly funded by industry, and the committees that control the use of drugs and devices are populated with members who receive financial support from the industry that benefits from the decisions they make. There's legitimate concern that this funding model may affect the process of drug approvals, with evidence that committee members who have ties to a drug's sponsor are more likely to vote for approval of that drug.

Good examples of regulatory control exist, such as the Pharmaceutical Benefits and Medical Services advisory committees in Australia, government bodies with governance structures and memberships that aren't tied to industry. These also have strict conflict-of-interest policies.

Universities

Medical courses can only offer a finite amount of content, and there's considerable competition to occupy the available space. Newly graduated doctors cannot be expected to know everything there is to know, but there are two areas of medical education we consider to be priorities in addressing the problems of overtreatment and medical harm. Firstly, doctors should be trained in the methods and practice of science-based medicine so that they can fully understand the relative risks and benefits of their decisions. This training would also mean they routinely and accurately appraise new information that becomes available and incorporate it into their practice if appropriate. This might mean doing things differently or not doing them at all. Secondly, they should be trained in how to communicate with patients, as outlined in chapter 4.

For many universities, a medical school is a source of income, sometimes subsidising other, less lucrative faculties. The cost of medical training can result in significant debt for doctors once they enter practice, indirectly driving up the costs of care and the incentive for doctors to provide more treatment. The average education debt for US medical graduates is just short of $200 000. Often, more debt is required to establish a practice, which makes it hard for doctors not to focus on the generation of income as a priority.

We were both lucky to have been trained in an era in Australia when higher education was free, and we feel that this has given us an obligation to public service. Although our country now has a fee-based system, it's possible for students to complete their education without private debt. The government carries the debt, and only recovers that debt when the debtor is earning above a certain threshold, after which time the loan is gradually repaid by deductions from wages.

In recognition of the need to prepare future doctors to practise environmentally sustainable health care, a collaboration of Australasian medical schools and medical student associations recently produced a resource to facilitate inclusion of the environment as a determinant of health in medical curricula. Many universities have also established planetary health departments, which will support much needed further research into the environmental effects of health care and how they can best be addressed.

* * *

Patients, doctors, the media, government, insurers and other stakeholders can all help to make medicine more effective, less harmful and cheaper. But many of the actions outlined above rely on accurate assessment of the effectiveness, harms and overall value of medical care. Most of all, however, the public, doctors and governments should all be aware of the problems and perverse incentives in the system, and acknowledge that things are not right – that we're wasting money and harming people. We live in a system where one approved drug can be widely adopted into clinical practice and kill tens of thousands of people, and barely anyone in the public know's about it. Medicine has been accused of being the third leading cause of death, and there's virtually no reaction beyond a shrug of the shoulders.

Many people dismiss data about medical harms as the price we pay for the rich rewards of modern medicine, but many of these harms are entirely preventable and therefore should not be dismissed as inevitable. We all need to start asking questions that challenge the status quo. No single solution can work in isolation. All parts of the complex system of health care need to be working in harmony to improve health, not just health care.

References and further reading

Introduction

Brownlee S, Chalkidou K, Doust J et al., 'Evidence for overuse of medical services around the world', *Lancet*, 2017, vol. 390, no. 10090, pp. 156–68

Institute of Medicine (US) Committee on Quality of Health Care in America, Kohn LT, Corrigan JM, Donaldson MS (eds), *To Err Is Human: Building a Safer Health System*, National Academies Press, Washington, DC, 2000, <https://doi.org/10.17226/9728>

Taber JM, Leyva B, Persoskie A, 'Why do people avoid medical care? A qualitative study using national data', *Journal of General Internal Medicine*, 2015, vol. 30, pp. 290–97

Kuehn BM, 'Shifting hydroxychloroquine patterns raise concern', *JAMA*, 2020, vol. 324, p. 1600

Australian Government Department of Health, 'Pete Evans' company fined for alleged COVID-19 advertising breaches', Therapeutic Goods Administration, 24 April 2020, <www.tga.gov.au/media-release/pete-evans-company-fined-alleged-covid-19-advertising-breaches>

Australian Government Department of Health, 'SGC products fined $63,000 for alleged unlawful advertising on "Dr Ageless" website in relation to COVID-19', Therapeutic Goods Administration, 31 July 2020, <www.tga.gov.au/media-release/sgc-products-fined-63000-alleged-unlawful-advertising-dr-ageless-website-relation-covid-19>

Thien F, Beggs PJ, Csutoros D et al., 'The Melbourne epidemic thunderstorm asthma event 2016: an investigation of environmental triggers, effect on health services, and patient risk factors', *Lancet Planet Health*, 2018, vol. 2, no. 6, pp. e255–63

Duckett S, Mackey W, Stobart A, 'The health effects of the 2019–20 bushfires: submission to the Royal Commission into National Natural Disaster Arrangements', Grattan Institute, 2020, <https://grattan.edu.au/wp-content/uploads/2020/04/Grattan-Institute-submission-to-Royal-Commission.pdf>

Malik A, Lenzen M, McAlister S, McGain F, 'The carbon footprint of Australian health care', *Lancet Planet Earth*, 2018, vol. 2, no. 1, pp. e27–35

1 First, do no harm

Walton M, 'Deep sleep therapy and Chelmsford Private Hospital: have we learnt anything?', *Australasian Psychiatry*, 2013, vol. 21, no. 3, pp. 206–12

Pols H, 'The Chelmsford scandal – reflection on physicians doing wrong', *Australasian Psychiatry*, 2013, vol. 21, no. 3, pp. 216–19

New South Wales (Slattery JP), *Report of the Royal Commission into Deep Sleep Therapy*, 14 vols, Government Printing Service, Sydney, 1990

'Chelmsford doctors trying to "rewrite history" lose defamation case against publisher', *The Guardian*, 25 November 2020, <www.theguardian.com/australia-news/2020/nov/25/chelmsford-doctors-trying-to-rewrite-history-lose-defamation-case-against-publisher>

Prasad V, Vandross A, Toomey C et al., 'A decade of reversal: an analysis of 146 contradicted medical practices', *Mayo Clinic Proceedings*, 2013, vol. 88, no. 8, pp. 790–98

Gerstein HC, Miller ME, Byington RP, et al., Action to Control Cardiovascular Risk in Diabetes Study Group. 'Effects of intensive glucose lowering in type 2 diabetes', N Engl J Med, 2008, vol. 358, no. 24, pp. 2545–2559

Patel A, MacMahon S, Chalmers J, et al., ADVANCE Collaborative Group. 'Intensive blood glucose control and vascular outcomes in patients with type 2 diabetes', N Engl J Med, 2008, vol. 358, no. 24, pp. 2560–2572

Grufferman S, Kim SYS, 'Clinical epidemiology defined', *New England Journal of Medicine*, 1984, vol. 311, pp. 541–42

Krogsbøll LT, Jørgensen KJ, Grønhøj Larsen C, Gøtzsche PC, 'General health checks in adults for reducing morbidity and mortality from disease', *Cochrane Database of Systematic Reviews*, 2012, issue 10, article no. CD009009

Institute of Medicine (US) Committee on Quality of Health Care in America, Kohn LT, Corrigan JM, Donaldson MS (eds), *To Err is Human: Building a Safer Health System*, National Academies Press, Washington, DC, 2000, <https://doi.org/10.17226/9728>

Institute of Medicine, Committee on the Learning Health Care System in America, Smith M, Saunders R, Stuckhardt L, McGinnis JM (eds), *Best Care at Lower Cost: The Path to Continuously Learning Health Care in America*, National Academies Press, Washington, DC, 2013, <www.nap.edu/catalog/13444/best-care-at-lower-cost-the-path-to-continuously-learning>

Wilson RM, Runciman WB, Gibberd RW et al., 'The Quality in Australian Health Care Study', *Medical Journal of Australia*, 1995, vol. 163, pp. 458–71

De Vries EN, Ramrattan MA, Smorenburg SM et al., 'The incidence and nature of in-hospital adverse events: a systematic review', *BMJ Quality and Safety*, 2008, vol. 17, pp. 216–23

Rafter N, Hickey A, Conroy RM et al., 'The Irish National Adverse Events Study (INAES): the frequency and nature of adverse events in Irish hospitals – a retrospective record review study', *BMJ Quality and Safety*, 2017, vol. 26:1, pp. 11–19

Wilson RM, Michel P, Olsen S et al., 'Patient safety in developing countries: retrospective estimation of scale and nature of harm to patients in hospital', *BMJ*, 2012, vol. 344, article no. e832

Slawomirski L, Auraaen A, Klazinga N, *The Economics of Patient Safety: Strengthening a Value-based Approach to Reducing Patient Harm at National Level*, OECD, Paris, 2017, <www.oecd.org/els/health-systems/The-economics-of-patient-safety-March-2017.pdf>

Davis P, Roy Lay-Yee R, Briant R et al., 'Adverse events in New Zealand public hospitals I: occurrence and impact', Occasional Paper no. 3, New Zealand Ministry of Health, Wellington, 2001, <www.health.govt.nz/system/files/documents/publications/adverseevents.pdf>

NORC at the University of Chicago and IHI/NPSF Lucian Leape Institute, *Americans' Experiences with Medical Errors and Views on Patient Safety*, Institute for Healthcare Improvement and NORC at the University of Chicago, Cambridge, MA, 2017, <www.ihi.org/about/news/Documents/IHI_NPSF_NORC_Patient_Safety_Survey_2017_Final_Report.pdf>

Korenstein D, Harris R, Elshaug AG et al., 'To expand the evidence base about harms from tests and treatments', *Journal of General Internal Medicine*, 2021

Louis PCA, 'Researches on the effects of blood-letting in some inflammatory diseases, and on the influence of tartarised antimony and vesication in pneumonitis', *American Journal of the Medical Sciences*, 1836, vol. 18, pp. 102–11

Milne I, Chalmers I, 'Alexander Lesassier Hamilton's 1816 report of a controlled trial of bloodletting', *Journal of the Royal Society of Medicine*, 2015, vol. 10, no. 2, pp. 68–60

Greenwood M., 'Louis and the numerical method', *The Medical Dictator and Other Biographical Studies*, London: Williams & Northgate, 1936, pp. 123–41

Stubbs JW, 'Sharing knowledge is part of a modern Hippocratic Oath', President's Message, American College of Physicians Internist, June 2009, <https://acpinternist.org/archives/2009/06/presidents.htm>

McVean A, 'The history of hysteria', Office for Science and Society, McGill University, 31 July 2017, <www.mcgill.ca/oss/article/history-quackery/history-hysteria>

Warner JH, 'Attitudes to foreign knowledge', *The Therapeutic Perspective: Medical Practice, Knowledge, and Identity in America, 1820–1885*, Harvard University Press, Cambridge, MA, 1986, pp. 185–206

Tan SY, Yip A, 'António Egas Moniz (1874–1955): lobotomy pioneer and Nobel laureate', *Singapore Medical Journal*, 2014, vol. 55, pp. 175–76

Rangachari PK, 'Evidence-based medicine: old French wine with a new Canadian label?', *Journal of the Royal Society of Medicine*, 1997, vol. 90, pp. 280–84

Brennan TA, Mello MM, 'The controversy over high-dose chemotherapy with autologous bone marrow transplant for breast cancer', *Health Affairs*, 2001, vol. 20, no. 5, pp. 101–17

Farquhar C, Marjoribanks J, Lethaby A, Azhar M, 'High-dose chemotherapy and autologous bone marrow or stem cell transplantation versus conventional chemotherapy for women with early poor prognosis breast cancer', *Cochrane Database of Systematic Reviews*, 2016, issue 5, article no. CD003139

Rettig RA, Jacobson PD, Farquhar CM, Aubry WM, *False Hope: Bone Marrow Transplantation for Breast Cancer*, Oxford University Press, New York, 2007

Bjelakovic G, Nikolova D, Gluud LL et al., 'Antioxidant supplements for prevention of mortality in healthy participants and patients with various diseases', *Cochrane Database of Systematic Reviews*, 2012, issue 3, article no. CD007176

Vargesson N, 'Thalidomide-induced teratogenesis: history and mechanisms. Birth Defects Research Part C', *Embryo Today*, 2015, vol. 105, pp. 140–56

Watts G, 'Frances Oldham Kelsey', *Lancet*, 2005, vol. 386, no. 10001, p. 1334

Vianna FSL, Lopez-Camelo JS, Leite JCL, 'Epidemiological surveillance of birth defects compatible with thalidomide embryopathy in Brazil', *PLOS ONE*, vol. 6, article no. e21735

Goetzsche P, *Deadly Medicines and Organised Crime: How Big Pharma Has Corrupted Healthcare*, CRC Press, London, 2013

References and further reading

Rosen CJ, 'The Rosiglitazone story – lessons from an FDA advisory committee meeting', *New England Journal of Medicine*, 2007, vol. 357, pp. 844–46

Rosen CJ, 'Revisiting the Rosiglitazone story – lessons learned', *New England Journal of Medicine*, 2010, vol. 363, pp. 803–806

Pantillo K, 'Accuracy of emergency nurses in assessment of patients' pain', *Pain Management Nursing*, 2003, vol. 4, no. 4, pp. 171–75

Lipman AG, 'Pain as a human right: the 2004 Global Day Against Pain', *Journal of Pain, Palliative Care and Pharmacotherapy*, 2005, vol. 19, no. 3, pp. 85–100

Gart M, 'Pain is not the fifth vital sign', *Medical Economics*, 20 May 2017, <www.medicaleconomics.com/medical-economics-blog/pain-not-fifth-vital-sign>

Chaparro EL, Furlan AD, Deshpande A et al., 'Opioids compared to placebo or other treatments for chronic low-back pain', *Cochrane Database of Systematic Reviews*, 2013, issue 8, article no. CD004959

Centers for Disease Control and Prevention, 'US opioid dispensing rate maps', 5 March 2020, <www.cdc.gov/drugoverdose/maps/rxrate-maps.html>

National Institute on Drug Abuse, 'Opioid overdose crisis', 27 May 2020, <www.drugabuse.gov/drug-topics/opioids/opioid-overdose-crisis>

Galofaro C, Schmall E, 'Far from U.S. epidemic, "the other opioid crisis" rages in vulnerable countries', *Los Angeles Times*, 13 December 2019, <www.latimes.com/world-nation/story/2019-12-13/safer-opioid-has-sparked-a-crisis-in-vulnerable-countries>

Blanch B, Pearson SA, Haber PS, 'An overview of the patterns of prescription opioid use, costs and related harms in Australia', *British Journal of Clinical Pharmacology*, 2014, vol. 78, no. 5, pp. 1159–66

Davis CS, 'The Purdue Pharma Opioid Settlement – accountability, or just the cost of doing business?', *New England Journal of Medicine*, 2021, vol. 384, no. 2, pp. 97–99

Keefe PR, 'Empire of pain: the Sackler family's ruthless promotion of opioids generated billions of dollars and millions of addicts', *New Yorker*, 30 October 2017

Keefe PR, 'The Sackler family's plan to keep its billions', *New Yorker*, 4 October 2020

Pratt M, Stevens A, Thuku M et al., 'Benefits and harms of medical cannabis: a scoping review of systematic reviews', *Systematic Reviews*, 2019, vol. 8, article no. 320

Farrell M, Buchbinder R, Hall W, 'Should doctors prescribe cannabinoids?', *BMJ*, 2014, vol. 348, article no. g2737

Hoffmann TC, Del Mar C, 'Patients' expectations of the benefits and harms of treatments, screening, and tests: a systematic review', *JAMA Internal Medicine*, 2015, vol. 175, no. 2, pp. 274–86

Hoffmann TC, Del Mar C, 'Clinicians' expectations of the benefits and harms of treatments, screening, and tests: a systematic review', *JAMA Internal Medicine*, 2017, vol. 177, no. 3, pp. 407–19

Buchbinder R, Bourne A, 'Content analysis of consumer information about knee arthroscopy in Australia', *Australian and New Zealand Journal of Surgery*, 2018, vol. 88, no. 4, pp. 346–53

Sheetz KH, Dimick JB, 'Is it time for safeguards in the adoption of robotic surgery?', *JAMA*, 2019, vol. 321, no. 20, pp. 1971–72

Anand R, Graves SE, de Steiger RN et al., 'What is the benefit of introducing new hip and knee prostheses?' *Journal of Bone and Joint Surgery* (American), 2001, vol. 93, supplement no. 3, pp. 51–54

Harris IA, Harris AM, Adie S et al., 'Discordance between patient and surgeon satisfaction after total joint arthroplasty', *Journal of Arthroplasty*, 2013, vol. 28, no. 5, pp. 722–27

Harris IA, Dao ATT, Young JM et al., 'Predictors of patient and surgeon satisfaction after orthopaedic trauma', *Injury*, 2009, vol. 40, no. 4, pp. 377–84

Courtney D, Huseyin N, Evrim G et al., 'Availability of evidence of benefits on overall survival and quality of life of cancer drugs approved by European Medicines Agency: retrospective cohort study of drug approvals 2009–13', *BMJ*, 2017, vol. 359, article no. j4530

Mailankody S, Prasad V, 'Overall survival in cancer drug trials as a new surrogate end point for overall survival in the real world', *JAMA Oncology*, 2017, vol. 3, no. 7, pp. 889–90

Chalmers I, Glasziou P, 'Avoidable waste in the production and reporting of research evidence', *Lancet*, 2009, vol. 374, no. 9683, pp. 86–89

Cilo CM, Larson EB, 'Exploring the harmful effects of healthcare', *JAMA*, 2009, vol. 302, pp. 89–89

Illich I, *Limits to Medicine. Medical Nemesis: The Expropriation of Health*, Marion Boyars, New York, 1995

Mackary MA, Daniel M, 'Medical error – the third leading cause of death in the US', *BMJ*, 2016, vol. 353, article no. i2139

Prasad V, Cifu A, Ioannidis JP, 'Reversals of established medical practices evidence to abandon ship', *JAMA*, 2012, vol.. 307, pp. 37–38

Epstein D, 'When evidence says no, but doctors say yes', *The Atlantic*, 22 February 2017, <www.theatlantic.com/health/archive/2017/02/when-evidence-says-no-but-doctors-say-yes/517368>

James JT, 'A new, evidence-based estimate of patient harms associated with hospital care', *Journal of Patient Safety*, 2013, vol. 9, no. 3, pp. 122–28

Davis P, Roy Lay-Yee R, Briant R, 'Adverse events in New Zealand public hospitals I: occurrence and impact', *New Zealand Medical Journal*, 2002, vol. 115, no. 1167, article no. U271

Leape LL, Shore MM, Dienstag JL et al., 'Perspective: a culture of respect, part 1: the nature and causes of disrespectful behavior by physicians', *Academic Medicine*, 2012, vol. 87, no. 7, pp. 845–52

Baker GR, Norton P, 'Addressing the effects of adverse events: study provides insights into patient safety at Canadian hospitals', *Healthcare Quarterly*, 2004, vol. 7, no. 4, pp. 20–21

Jha AK, Larizgoitia I, Audera-Lopez C et al., 'The global burden of unsafe medical care: analytic modelling of observational studies', *BMJ Quality and Safety*, 2013, vol. 22, pp. 809–15

Slawomirski L, Auraaen A, Klazinga N, 'The Economics of Patient Safety: Strengthening a Value-based Approach to Reducing Patient Harm at National Level', OECD, Paris, 2017, <www.oecd.org/els/health-systems/The-economics-of-patient-safety-March-2017.pdf>

Lyu H, Cooper MA, Mayer-Blackwell BBS et al., 'Medical harm: patient perceptions and follow-up actions', *Journal of Patient Safety*, 2017, vol. 13, no. 4, pp. 199–201

Lyu H, Xu T, Brotman D et al., 'Overtreatment in the United States', *PLOS ONE*, 2017, vol. 12, no. 9, article no. e0181970

Jena AB, Prasad V, Goldman DP, Romley J, 'Mortality and treatment patterns among patients hospitalized with acute cardiovascular conditions during dates of national cardiology meetings', *JAMA Internal Medicine*, 2015, vol. 175, no. 2, pp. 237–44

Wang L, Hong PJ, May C et al., 'Medical cannabis for chronic pain: a systematic review and meta-analysis of randomized clinical trials', *BMJ*, 2021, vol. XX, article no. XX

The National Institute for Health and Care Excellence (NICE), Cannabis-based Medicinal Products: [B] Evidence Review for Chronic Pain, NICE Guideline NG144, NICE, London, 2019, <www.nice.org.uk/guidance/ng144/evidence/b-chronic-pain-pdf-6963831759>

Kim C, Prasad V, 'Strength of validation for surrogate end points used in the US Food and Drug Administration's approval of oncology drugs', *Mayo Clin Proc* 2016, vol, 91, pp. 713-25

Lenzen M, Malik A, Li M et al., 'The environmental footprint of health care: a global assessment', *Lancet Planet Health*, 2020, vol. 4, no. 7, pp. e271–79

Costello A, Abbas M, Allen A et al., 'Managing the health effects of climate change: *Lancet* and University College London Institute for Global Health Commission', *Lancet*, 2009, vol. 373, no. 9676, pp. 1693–33

McAlister S, Ou Y, Neff E et al., 'The environmental footprint of morphine: a life cycle assessment from opium poppy farming to the packaged drug', *BMJ Open*, 2016, vol. 6, article no. e013302

Thiel CL, Eckelman MJ, Guido R et al., 'Environmental impacts of surgical procedures: life cycle assessment of hysterectomy in the US', *Environmental Science and Technology*, 2015, vol. 49, pp. 1779–86

Sherman J, Le C, Lamers V, Eckelman M, 'Life cycle greenhouse gas emissions of anesthetic drugs', *Anesthesia and Analgesia*, 2012, vol. 114, pp. 1086–90

McAlister S, Barratt AL, Bell KJL et al., 'The carbon footprint of pathology testing', *Medical Journal of Australia*, 2020, vol. 212, no. 8, pp. 377–82

McGain F, Blashki GA, Moon KP, Armstrong FM, 'Mandating sustainability in Australian hospitals', *Medical Journal of Australia*, 2009, vol. 190, no. 12, pp. 719–20

2 Science matters

Harris IA, Sidhu V, Mittal R, Adie S, 'Surgery for chronic musculoskeletal pain: the question of evidence', *Pain*, 2020, vol. 161, no. 9, supplement no. 1, pp. S95–103

McGlynn EA, Asch SM, Adams J et al., 'The quality of health care delivered to adults in the United States', *New England Journal of Medicine*, 2003, vol. 348, pp. 2635–45

Runciman WB, Hunt TD, Hannaford NA et al., 'CareTrack: assessing the appropriateness of health care delivery in Australia', *Medical Journal of Australia*, 2012, vol. 197, no. 2, pp. 100–105

Glasziou P, Haynes B, 'The paths from research to improved health outcomes', *BMJ Evidence-Based Medicine*, 2005, vol. 10, pp. 4–7

Morris ZS, Wooding S, Grant J, 'The answer is 17 years, what is the question: understanding time lags in translational research', *Journal of the Royal Society of Medicine*, 2011, vol. 104, no. 12, pp. 510–20

World Health Organization, *Bridging the 'Know–Do' Gap:. Meeting on Knowledge Translation in Global Health, 10–12 October 2005*, WHO, Geneva, 2006

Gaynes RP, *Germ Theory: Medical Pioneers in Infectious Diseases*, John Wiley & Sons, New York, 2011

World Health Organization, *Guidelines on Core Components of Infection Prevention and Control Programmes at the National and Acute Health Care Facility Level*, WHO, Geneva, 2016

Grayson ML, Russo PL, Cruickshank M et al., 'Outcomes from the first 2 years of the Australian National Hand Hygiene Initiative', *Medical Journal of Australia*, 2011, vol. 195, no. 10, pp. 615–19

Moore LD, Robbins G, Quinn J, Arbogast JW, 'The impact of COVID-19 pandemic on hand hygiene performance in hospitals', *American Journal of Infection Control*, 2020, vol. 49, no. 1, pp. 30–33

Green LW, 'Making research relevant: if it is an evidence-based practice, where's the practice-based evidence?', *Family Practice*, 2008, vol. 25, supplement no. 1, pp. i20–24

Balas EA, Biren SA, 'Managing clinical knowledge for health care improvement', *Yearbook of Medical Informatics*, 2000, vol. 1, pp. 65–70

Mickan S, Burls A, Glasziou P, 'Patterns of "leakage" in the utilisation of clinical guidelines: a systematic review', *Postgraduate Medical Journal*, 2011, vol. 87, pp. 670–79

Cabana MD, Rand CS, Powe NR et al., 'Why don't physicians follow clinical practice guidelines? A framework for improvement', *JAMA*, 1999, vol. 282, no. 15, pp. 1458–65

Lantin B, 'A miracle for bone fractures', *Telegraph* (London), 2 April 2003, <www.telegraph.co.uk/news/health/elder/3301063/A-miracle-for-bone-fractures.html>

Buchbinder R, Osborne R, 'Vertebroplasty: a promising but as yet unproven intervention for painful osteoporotic spinal fractures', *Medical Journal of Australia*, 2016, vol. 185, no. 7, pp. 351–52

Buchbinder R, Osborne RH, Ebeling PR et al., 'A randomized trial of vertebroplasty for painful osteoporotic vertebral fractures', *New England Journal of Medicine*, 2009, vol. 361, pp. 557–68

Kallmes DF, Comstock BA, Heagerty PJ et al., 'A randomized trial of vertebroplasty for osteoporotic spinal fractures', *New England Journal of Medicine*, 2009, vol. 361, pp. 569–79

Buchbinder R, Johnston R, Rischin KJ et al., 'Percutaneous vertebroplasty for osteoporotic vertebral compression fracture', *Cochrane Database of Systematic Reviews*, 2018, issue 11, article no. CD006349

Buchbinder R, Busija L, 'Why we should stop performing vertebroplasties', *Internal Medicine Journal*, 2019, vol. 49, pp. 1367–71

Carragee E, 'The vertebroplasty affair: the mysterious case of the disappearing effect size', *Spine Journal*, 2010, vol. 10, no. 3, pp. 191–92

Wulff KC, Miller FG, Pearson SD, 'Can coverage be rescinded when negative trial results threaten a popular procedure? The ongoing saga of vertebroplasty', *Health Affairs*, 2011, vol. 30, no. 12, pp. 2269–76

Pinsker J, 'The covert world of people trying to edit Wikipedia – for pay', *The Atlantic*, 11 August 2015, <www.theatlantic.com/business/archive/2015/08/wikipedia-editors-for-pay/393926>

Hayes MJ, Kaestner V, Mailankody S, Prasad V, 'Most medical practices are not parachutes: a citation analysis of practices felt by biomedical authors to be analogous to parachutes', *Canadian Medical Association Journal Open*, 2018, vol. 6, pp. E31–38

Carvalho C, Caetano JM, Cunha L et al., 'Open-label placebo treatment in chronic low back pain: a randomized controlled trial', *Pain*, 2016, vol. 157, pp. 2766–72

Wood L, Egger M, Gluud LL et al., 'Empirical evidence of bias in treatment effect estimates in controlled trials with different interventions and outcomes: meta-epidemiological study', *BMJ*, 2008, vol. 336, article no. 601

Siemieniuk RAC, Harris IA, Agoritsas T et al., 'Arthroscopic surgery for degenerative knee arthritis and meniscal tears: a clinical practice guideline', *BMJ*, 2017, vol. 357, article no. j1982

Vandvik PO, Lähdeoja T, Ardern C et al., 'Subacromial decompression surgery for adults with shoulder pain: a clinical practice guideline', *BMJ*, 2019, vol. 364, article no. l294

Karjalainen TV, Jain NB, Page CM et al., 'Subacromial decompression surgery for rotator cuff disease', *Cochrane Database of Systematic Reviews*, 2019, issue 1, article no CD005619

Karjalainen TV, Jain NB, Heikkinen H et al., 'Surgery for rotator cuff tears', *Cochrane Database of Systematic Reviews*, 2019, issue 12, article no. CD013502

Gupta VK, Saini C, Oberoi M, Imran Nasir Md, 'Semmelweis reflex: an age-old prejudice', *World Neurosurgery*, 2020, vol. 136, pp. e119–25

Daube M, 'Targets and abuse: the price public health campaigners pay', *Medical Journal of Australia*, 2015, vol. 202, no. 6, pp. 294–96

Pincock S, 'Nobel Prize winners Robin Warren and Barry Marshall', *Lancet*, 2005, vol. 366, no. 9495, p. 1429

Laskas JM, 'Bennet Omalu, concussions, and the NFL: how one doctor changed football forever', *GQ*, 15 September 2009, <www.gq.com/story/nfl-players-brain-dementia-study-memory-concussions>

Laskas JM, *Concussion*, Random House, New York, 2015

Belson K, 'The concussion crisis in Australian Rules Football', *New York Times*, 26 September 2019

Gabriel SE, O'Fallon WM, Kurland LT et al., 'Risk of connective-tissue diseases and other disorders after breast implantation', *New England Journal of Medicine*, 1994, vol. 330, pp. 1697–1702

Angel M, *Science on Trial: The Clash of Medical Evidence and the Law in the Breast Implant Case*, W.W. Norton & Company, New York, 1996

Buchbinder R, Ptasznik R, Gordon J et al., 'Ultrasound-guided extracorporeal shock wave therapy for plantar fasciitis: a randomized controlled trial', *JAMA*, 2002, vol. 288, pp. 1364–72

Van der Weyden MB, 'Vertebroplasty, evidence and professional protest', *Medical Journal of Australia*, 2010, vol. 192, no. 6, pp. 301–302

Staples MP, Kallmes DF, Comstock BA et al., 'Effectiveness of vertebroplasty using individual patient data from two randomised placebo controlled trials: meta-analysis', *BMJ*, 2011, vol. 342, article no. d3952

Mann ME, *The Hockey Stick and the Climate Wars*, Columbia University Press, New York, 2012

Barratt A, Howard K, Irwig L, Salkeld G, Houssami N, 'Model of outcomes of screening mammography: information to support informed choices', *BMJ*, 2005, vol. 330, article no. 936

Johansson M, Hansson A, Brodersen J, 'Estimating overdiagnosis in screening for abdominal aortic aneurysm: could a change in smoking habits and lowered aortic diameter tip the balance of screening towards harm?', *BMJ*, 2015, vol. 350, article no. h825

Johansson M, Jørgensen KJ, Brodersen J, 'Harms of screening for abdominal aortic aneurysm: is there more to life than a 0·46% disease-specific mortality reduction?', *Lancet*, 2016, vol. 387, no. 10015, pp. 308–10

Buchbinder R, Harris I, 'Arthroscopy for osteoarthritis of the knee?', *Medical Journal of Australia*, 2012, vol. 197, no. 7, pp. 364–65

'Wasted', *Four Corners*, ABC, 28 September 2015, <www.abc.net.au/4corners/wasted-promo/6804372>

Fritz A, 'The confidence of the incompetent', *Financial Review*, 14 January 2019

Begley CG, Ellis LM, 'Drug development: raise standards for preclinical cancer research', *Nature*, 2012, vol. 483, pp. 531–33

Ioannidis JPA, 'Contradicted and initially stronger effects in highly cited clinical research', *JAMA*, 2005, vol. 294, no. 2, pp. 218–28

Prinz F, Schlange T, Asadullah K, 'Believe it or not: how much can we rely on published data on potential drug targets?', *Nature Reviews Drug Discovery*, 2011, vol. 10, article no. 712

Prasad V, Vandross A, Toomey C et al., 'A decade of reversal: an analysis of 146 contradicted medical practices', *Mayo Clinic Proceedings*, 2013, vol. 88, no. 8, pp. 790–98

3 Overtreatment

Kaiser AD, 'Results of tonsillectomy: a comparative study of twenty-two hundred tonsillectomized children with an equal number of controls three and ten years after operation', *JAMA*, 1930, vol. 95, no. 12, pp. 837–42

Washington Health Alliance, *First, Do No Harm: Calculating Health Care Waste in Washington State*, WHA, Seattle, 2018, <www.wacommunitycheckup.org/media/47156/2018-first-do-no-harm.pdf>

'Wasted', *Four Corners*, ABC, 28 September 2015, <www.abc.net.au/4corners/wasted-promo/6804372>

Brodersen J, Schwartz LM, Heneghan C et al., 'Overdiagnosis: what it is and what it isn't', *BMJ Evidence-Based Medicine*, 2018, vol. 23, pp. 1–3

BMJ, 'Too Much Medicine' series, <www.bmj.com/too-much-medicine>

JAMA Network, 'Less is More' series, <jamanetwork.com/collections/44045/less-is-more>

Journal of Hospital Medicine, 'Choosing Wisely: Things We Do for No Reason' series, <www.journalofhospitalmedicine.com/jhospmed/choosing-wisely-things-we-do-no-reason>

'National Action Plan: Initial Statement to underpin the development of a National Action Plan to Prevent Overdiagnosis and Overtreatment in Australia', <www.wiserhealthcare.org.au/national-action-plan>

Lyu H, Xu T, Brotman D et al., 'Overtreatment in the United States', *PLOS ONE*, 2017, vol. 12, no. 9, article no. e0181970

Institute of Medicine (US) Committee on Quality of Health Care in America; Kohn LT, Corrigan JM, Donaldson MS (eds), *To Err is Human: Building a Safer Health System*, National Academies Press, Washington, DC, 2000

Landrigan CP, Parry GJ, Bones CB et al., 'Temporal trends in rates of patient harm resulting from medical care', *New England Journal of Medicine*, 2010, vol. 363, no. 22, pp. 2124–34

References and further reading

Scott IA, 'Audit-based measures of overuse of medical care in Australian hospital practice', *Internal Medicine Journal*, 2019, vol. 49, no. 7, pp. 893–904

Hoffmann TC, Del Mar C, 'Clinicians' expectations of the benefits and harms of treatments, screening, and tests: a systematic review', *JAMA Internal Medicine*, 2017, vol. 177, no. 3, pp. 407–19

Committee on the Learning Health Care System in America; Institute of Medicine; Smith M, Saunders R, Stuckhardt L et al. (eds), *Best Care at Lower Cost: The Path to Continuously Learning Health Care in America*, National Academies Press, Washington, DC, 2013

Brownlee S, Chalkidou K, Doust J et al., 'Evidence for overuse of medical services around the world', *Lancet*, 2017, vol. 390, no. 10090, pp. 156–68

Boden WE, O'Rourke RA, Teo KK et al. for the COURAGE Trial Investigators, 'Optimal medical therapy with or without PCI for stable coronary disease', *New England Journal of Medicine*, 2007, vol. 356, pp. 1503–16

Sedlis SP, Hartigan PM, Teo KK et al. for the COURAGE Trial Investigators, 'Effect of PCI on long-term survival in patients with stable ischemic heart disease', *New England Journal of Medicine*, 2015, vol. 373, pp. 1937–46

Al-Lamee R, Thompson D, Dehbi H-M et al., 'Percutaneous coronary intervention in stable angina (ORBITA): a double-blind, randomised controlled trial', *Lancet*, 2018, vol. 391, no. 10115, pp. 31–40

Maron DJ, Hochman JS, Reynolds HR et al., 'Initial invasive or conservative strategy for stable coronary disease', *New England Journal of Medicine*, 2020, vol. 382, pp. 1395–1407

Salazar JW, Redberg RF, 'Two remedies for inappropriate percutaneous coronary intervention – closing the gap between evidence and practice', *JAMA Internal Medicine*, 2020, no. 1, pp. 1536–37

Australian Commission on Safety and Quality in Health Care and National Health Performance Authority, *Australian Atlas of Healthcare Variation*, ACSQHC, Sydney, 2015, <www.safetyandquality.gov.au/our-work/healthcare-variation/atlas-2015>

Australian Commission on Safety and Quality in Health Care and Australian Institute of Health and Welfare, *The Second Australian Atlas of Healthcare Variation*, ACSQHC, Sydney, 2017, <www.safetyandquality.gov.au/our-work/healthcare-variation/atlas-2017>

Australian Commission on Safety and Quality in Health Care and Australian Institute of Health and Welfare, *The Third Australian Atlas of Healthcare Variation*, 2018, ACSQHC, Sydney, <www.safetyandquality.gov.au/our-work/healthcare-variation/third-atlas-2018>

Försth P, Ólafsson G, Carlsson T et al., 'A randomized, controlled trial of fusion surgery for lumbar spinal stenosis', *New England Journal of Medicine*, 2016, vol. 374, no. 15, pp. 1413–23

Mello MM, Chandra A, Gawande A, Studdert DM, 'National costs of the medical liability system', *Health Affairs*, 2010, vol. 29, no. 9, pp. 1569–77

Naugler C, 'More than half of abnormal results from laboratory tests ordered by family physicians could be false-positive', *Canadian Family Physician*, 2018, vol. 64, pp. 202–203

Rozbroj T, Haas R, O'Connor D et al., 'A thematic meta-synthesis of qualitative studies investigating how patients and the public understand overtesting and overdiagnosis', *Social Science & Medicine*, 2021, manuscript under review

Franz EW, Bentley JN, Yee PPS et al., 'Patient misconceptions concerning lumbar spondylosis diagnosis and treatment', *Journal of Neurosurgery Spine*, 2015, vol. 22, no. 5, pp. 496–502

Haas R, Buchbinder R, 'Weighing up the potential benefits and harms of comprehensive full body health checks', Croakey, 24 August 2020, <www.croakey.org/weighing-up-the-potential-benefits-and-harms-of-comprehensive-full-body-health-checks>

Krogsbøll LT, Jørgensen KJ, Gøtzsche PC, 'General health checks in adults for reducing morbidity and mortality from disease', Cochrane Database of Systematic Reviews, 2019, Issue 1, article no. CD009009

Carter SM, Doust J, Degeling C et al., 'A definition and ethical evaluation of overdiagnosis: response to commentaries', *Journal of Medical Ethics*, 2016, vol. 42, pp. 722–24

Wiener RS, Schwartz LM, Woloshin S, 'When a test is too good: how CT pulmonary angiograms find pulmonary emboli that do not need to be found', *BMJ*, 2013, vol. 347, article no. f3368

Wennberg J, 'Commentary: a debt of gratitude to J. Alison Glover', *International Journal of Epidemiology*, 2008, vol. 37, no. 1, pp. 26–29

Hutchinson BD, Navin P, Marom EM, Truong MT, Bruzzi JF, 'Overdiagnosis in pulmonary embolism by pulmonary CT angiography', *American Journal of Roentgenology*, 2015, vol. 205, no. 2, pp. 837–42

Lenza M, Buchbinder R, Staples MP et al., 'Second opinion for degenerative spinal conditions: an option or a necessity? A prospective observational study', *BMC Musculoskeletal Disorders*, 2017, vol. 18, p. 354

Glasziou P, Jones M, Pathirana T, Barratt A, Bell K, 'Estimating the magnitude of cancer overdiagnosis in Australia', *Medical Journal of Australia*, 2020, vol. 212, pp. 163–68

Gøtzsche PC, Jørgensen KJ, 'Screening for breast cancer with mammography', Cochrane Database of Systematic Reviews, 2013, Issue 6, article no. CD001877

Cancer Australia, *Report on the Lung Cancer Screening Enquiry*, Cancer Australia, Sydney, 2020

Menon U, Gentry-Maharaj A, Burnell M et al., 'Ovarian cancer population screening and mortality after long-term follow-up in the UK Collaborative Trial of Ovarian Cancer Screening (UKCTOCS): a randomised controlled trial', *Lancet*, 2021, vol. 397, no. 10290, pp. 2182–93

Jacobs IJ, Menon U, Ryan A et al., 'Ovarian cancer screening and mortality in the UK Collaborative Trial of Ovarian Cancer Screening (UKCTOCS): a randomised controlled trial', *Lancet*, 2016, vol. 387, no. 10022, pp. 945–56

Bleyer A, Welch HG, 'Effect of three decades of screening mammography on breast-cancer incidence', *New England Journal of Medicine*, 2012, vol. 367, pp. 1998–2005

Ahn HS, Kim HJ, Welch HG, 'Korea's thyroid-cancer "epidemic" – screening and overdiagnosis', *New England Journal of Medicine*, 2014, vol. 371, pp. 1765–67

Tsubono Y, Hisamichi S, 'A halt to neuroblastoma screening in Japan', *New England Journal of Medicine*, 2004, vol. 350, pp. 2010–11

Ellison LM, Heaney JA, Birkmeyer JD, 'Trends in the use of radical prostatectomy for treatment of prostate cancer', *Effective Clinical Practice*, 1999, vol. 2, pp. 228–33

Fenton JJ, Weyrich MS, Durbin S et al., 'Prostate-specific antigen–based screening for prostate cancer: evidence report and systematic review for the US Preventive Services Task Force', *JAMA*, 2018, vol. 319, no. 18, pp. 1914–31

References and further reading

US Preventive Services Task Force, 'Screening for prostate cancer: US Preventive Services Task Force recommendation statement', *JAMA*, 2018, vol. 319, no. 18, pp. 1901–13

Ilic D, Neuberger MM, Djulbegovic M, Dahm P, 'Screening for prostate cancer', *Cochrane Database of Systematic Reviews*, 2013, issue 1, article no. CD004720

Allred DC, 'Ductal carcinoma in situ: terminology, classification, and natural history', *Journal of the National Cancer Institute Monographs*, 2010, vol. 2010, no. 41, pp. 134–38

Narod SA, Iqbal J, Giannakeas V, Sopik V, Sun P, 'Breast cancer mortality after a diagnosis of ductal carcinoma in situ', *JAMA Oncology*, 2015, vol. 1, no. 7, pp. 888–96

Barrio AV, Van Zee KJ, 'Controversies in the treatment of DCIS', *Annual Review of Medicine*, 2017, vol. 68, pp. 197–211

Sadate A, Occean BV, Beregi J-P et al., 'Systematic review and meta-analysis on the impact of lung cancer screening by low-dose computed tomography', *European Journal of Cancer*, 2020, vol. 134, pp. 107–14

Schwitzer G, 'How do journalist cover treatments, tests, products, and procedures? An evaluation of 500 stories', *PLOS Medicine*, 2008, vol. 5, no. 5, article no. e95

O'Keeffe M, Nickel B, Dakin T et al., 'Journalists' views on media coverage of medical tests and overdiagnosis: a qualitative study', *BMJ Open*, 2021, vol. 11, article no. e043991

Selvaraj S, Borkar DS, Prasad V, 'Media coverage of medical journals: do the best articles make the news?', *PLOS ONE*, 2014, vol. 9, no. 1, article no. e85355

Moynihan R, Medew J, 'Improving coverage of medical research in a changing media environment', *Canadian Medical Association Journal*, 2017, vol. 189, pp. E551–52

Li M, Chapman S, Agho K, Eastman CJ, 'Can even minimal news coverage influence consumer health-related behaviour?', *Health Education Research*, 2008, vol. 23, no. 3, pp. 543–48

Prasad V, Lenzer J, Newman DH, 'Why cancer screening has never been shown to "save lives" – and what we can do about it', *BMJ*, 2016, vol. 352, article no. h6080

Wilson J, Junger G, 'Principles and practice of screening for disease', Public Health Paper no. 34, World Health Organization, Geneva, 1968

Andermann A, Blancquart I, Beauchamp S, Déry V, 'Revisiting Wilson and Jungner in the genomic age: a review of screening criteria over the past 40 years', *Bulletin of the World Health Organization*, 2008, vol. 86, no. 4, pp. 317–19

Brinjikji W, Luetmer PH, Comstock BW et al., 'Systematic literature review of imaging features of spinal degeneration in asymptomatic populations', *American Journal of Neuroradiology*, 2015, vol. 36, pp. 2394–99

Maher C, O'Keeffe M, Buchbinder R, Harris I, 'Musculoskeletal healthcare: have we over-egged the pudding?', *International Journal of Rheumatic Disease*, 2019, vol. 22, no. 11, pp. 1957–60

Bell KJ, Doust J, Glasziou P et al., 'Recognizing the potential for overdiagnosis: are high-sensitivity cardiac troponin assays an example?', *Annals of Internal Medicine*, 2019, vol. 170, no. 4, pp. 1–4

Biller-Andorno N, Jüni P, 'Abolishing mammography screening programs? A view from the Swiss Medical Board', *New England Journal of Medicine*, 2014, vol. 370, no. 21, pp. 1965–67

267

Barratt A, Jørgensen KJ, Autier P, 'Reform of the National Screening Mammography Program in France', *JAMA Internal Medicine*, 2018, vol. 178, no. 2, pp. 177–78

Independent UK Panel on Breast Cancer Screening, 'The benefits and harms of breast cancer screening: an independent review', *Lancet*, 2012, vol. 380, no. 9855, pp. 1778–86

4 Warmth and sympathy

Holmes D, 'Mid Staffordshire scandal highlights NHS cultural crisis', *Lancet*, 2013, vol. 381, no. 9866, pp. 521–22

Singer T, Klimecki OM, 'Empathy and compassion', *Current Biology*, 2014, vol. 24, no. 18, pp. R875–78

Shelley BP, 'A value forgotten in doctoring: empathy', *Archives of Medical and Health Sciences*, 2015, vol. 3, pp. 169–73

Barsky AJ, 'The iatrogenic potential of the physician's words', *JAMA*, 2017, vol. 318, no. 24, pp. 2425–26

Kaptchuk TJ, Kelley JM, Conboy LA et al., 'Components of placebo effect: randomised controlled trial in patients with irritable bowel syndrome', *BMJ*, 2008, vol. 336, no. 7651, pp. 999–1003

Emanuel EJ, 'The status of end-of-life care in the United States: the glass is half full', *JAMA*, 2018, vol. 320, no. 3, pp. 239–41

Howick J, Moscrop A, Mebius A et al., 'Effects of empathic and positive communication in healthcare consultations: a systematic review and meta-analysis', *Journal of the Royal Society of Medicine*, 2018, vol. 111, no. 7, pp. 240–52

John M Kelley et al., 'Patient and practitioner influences on the placebo effect in irritable bowel syndrome', *Psychosomatic Medicine*, 2009, vol. 71, no. 7, p. 789

Patel S, Pelletier-Buli A, Smith S et al., 'Curricula for empathy and compassion training in medical education: a systematic review', *PLOS ONE*, vol. 14, no. 8, article no. e0221412

Young ME, Norman GR, Humphreys KR, 'The role of medical language in changing public perceptions of illness', *PLOS ONE*, 2008, vol. 3, no. 12, article no. e3875

Tulsky JA, Arnold RM, Alexander SC et al., 'Enhancing communication between oncologists and patients with a computer-based training program: a randomized trial', *Annals of Internal Medicine*, 2011, vol. 155, no. 9, pp. 593–601

Boodman SG, 'How to teach doctors empathy: "Being a good doctor requires an understanding of people, not just science"', *The Atlantic*, 15 March 2015, <www.theatlantic.com/health/archive/2015/03/how-to-teach-doctors-empathy/387784>

Coan JA, Schaefer HS, Davidson RJ, 'Lending a hand: social regulation of the neural response to threat', *Psychological Science*, 2006, vol. 17, no. 12, pp. 1032–39

Nickel B, Barratt A, Copp T et al., 'Words do matter: a systematic review on how different terminology for the same condition influences management preferences', *BMJ Open*, 2017, vol. 7, article no. e014129

Rosenkrantz AB, 'Differences in perceptions among radiologists, referring physicians, and patients regarding language for incidental findings reporting', *American Journal of Roentgenology*, 2017, vol. 208, no. 1, pp. 140–43

Bossen JKJ, Hageman MGJS, King JD, Ring DC, 'Does rewording MRI reports improve patient understanding and emotional response to a clinical report?', *Clinical Orthopaedics and Related Research*, 2013, vol. 471, no. 11, pp. 3637–44

References and further reading

Slade D, Manidis M, McGregor J et al., *Communicating in Hospital Emergency Departments*, Springer, Berlin, Heidelberg, 2015

Slade D, Scheeres H, Manidis M et al., 'Emergency communication: the discursive challenges facing emergency clinicians and patients in hospital emergency departments', *Discourse and Communication*, 2008, vol. 2, no. 3, pp. 271–98

Allegretti A, Borkan J, Reis S, Griffiths F, 'Paired interviews of shared experiences around chronic low back pain: classic mismatch between patients and their doctors', *Family Practice*, 2010, vol. 27, pp. 676–83

Stacey D, Légaré F, Lewis K et al., 'Decision aids for people facing health treatment or screening decisions', *Cochrane Database of Systematic Reviews*, 2017, issue 4, article no. CD001431

Huntington B, Kuhn N, 'Communication gaffes: a root cause of malpractice claims', *Proceedings* (Baylor University Medical Center), 2003, vol. 16, no. 2, pp. 157–61

Krouss M, Croft L, Morgan DJ, 'Physician understanding and ability to communicate harms and benefits of common medical treatments', *JAMA Internal Medicine*, 2016, vol. 176, no. 10, pp. 1565–67

Ubel PA, Angott AM, Zikmund-Fisher BJ, 'Physicians recommend different treatments for patients than they would choose for themselves', *Archives of Internal Medicine*, 2011, vol. 171, no. 7, pp. 630–34

Kachalia A, Kaufman SR, Boothman R et al., 'Liability claims and costs before and after implementation of a medical error disclosure program', *Annals of Internal Medicine*, 2010, vol. 153, pp. 213–21

Blake V, 'Medicine, the law, and conceptions of evidence', *AMA Journal of Ethics*, 2013, vol. 15, no. 1, pp. 46–50

Mello MM, Brennan TA, 'Deterrence of medical errors: theory and evidence for malpractice reform', *Texas Law Review*, 2002, vol. 50: 1595–1637

5 I know not

Bongers, PM Kremer AM, ter Laak J, 'Are psychosocial factors, risk factors for symptoms and signs of the shoulder, elbow, or hand/wrist?: A review of the epidemiological literature', *American Journal of Industrial Medicine*, 2002, vol. 41, no. 5, pp. 315–42

Lucire Y, *Constructing RSI*, UNSW Press, Sydney, 2004

Hadler NM, 'Industrial rheumatology: the Australian and New Zealand experiences with arm pain and back ache in the workplace', *Medical Journal of Australia*, 1986, vol. 144, pp. 191–95

Ferguson DA, '"RSI": putting the epidemic to rest', *Medical Journal of Australia*, 1987, vol. 147, pp. 213–14

Barton N, 'Repetitive strain disorder', *BMJ*, 1989, vol. 299, no. 6696, pp. 405–06

Hadler NM, 'Work-related disorders of the upper extremity part I: cumulative trauma disorders – a critical review', in NM Hadler, WB Bunn (eds), *Occupational Problems in Medical Practice*, Delacorte Press, New York, 1990, pp. 219–48

Semple JC, 'Tenosynovitis, repetitive strain injury, cumulative trauma disorder, and overuse syndrome et cetera', *Journal of Bone and Joint Surgery* (British), 1991, vol. 73, no. 4, pp. 536–38

Stevenson N, 'Autism doesn't have to be viewed as a disability or disorder', *The Guardian*, 16 July 2015, <www.theguardian.com/science/blog/2015/jul/16/autism-doesnt-have-to-be-viewed-as-a-disability-or-disorder>

Jordan R and Collins G (an exchange of letters), 'What's the point of the "autism" label?', *The Psychologist*, 2015, vol. 28, <thepsychologist.bps.org.uk/volume-28/march-2015/whats-point-autism-label>

Harris IA, 'The association between compensation and outcome after injury', PhD thesis, University of Sydney, 2006, <http://hdl.handle.net/2123/1892>

Hartvigsen J, Hoy D, Smeets R et al., for the *Lancet* Low Back Pain Series Working Group, 'What low back pain is and why we need to pay attention', *Lancet*, 2018, vol. 391, no. 10137, pp. 2356–67

Foster NE, Koes B, Chou R et al., 'Prevention and treatment of low back pain: evidence, challenges, and promising directions', *Lancet*, 2018, vol. 391, no. 10137, pp. 2368–83

Buchbinder R, van Tulder M, Öberg B et al., 'Low back pain: a call for action', *Lancet*, 2018, vol. 391, no. 10137, pp. 2384–88

Buchbinder R, Maher C, Underwood M, Hartvigsen J, 'The *Lancet* series call to action to reduce low value care for low back pain: an update', *Pain*, 2020, vol. 161, pp. S57–64

Artus M, van der Windt DA, Jordan KP, Hay EM, 'Low back pain symptoms show a similar pattern of improvement following a wide range of primary care treatments: a systematic review of randomized clinical trials', *Rheumatology*, 2010, vol. 49, no. 12, pp. 2346–56

Buchbinder R, Batterham R, Eldsworth G et al., 'A validity-driven approach to the understanding of the personal and societal burden of low back pain: development of a conceptual and measurement model', *Arthritis Research and Therapy*, 2011, vol. 13, article no. R152

Williams CM, Maher CG, Latimer J et al., 'Efficacy of paracetamol for acute low-back pain: a double-blind, randomised controlled trial', *Lancet*, 2014, vol. 384, no. 9954, pp. 1586–96

Chou R, Wagner J, Ahmed AY et al., *Treatments for Acute Pain: A Systematic Review*, Comparative Effectiveness Review no. 240, AHRQ Publication No. 20(21)-EHC006, Agency for Healthcare Research and Quality, Rockville, MD, 2020

Enke O, New HA, New CH et al., 'Anticonvulsants in the treatment of low back pain and lumbar radicular pain: a systematic review and meta-analysis', *Canadian Medical Association Journal*, 2018, vol. 190, pp. E786–93

Gomes T, Greaves S, van den Brink W et al., 'Pregabalin and the risk for opioid-related death: a nested case control study', *Annals of Internal Medicine*, 2018, vol. 169, no. 10, pp. 732–34

Buchbinder R, Jolley D, Wyatt M, 'Population based intervention to change back pain beliefs and disability: three part evaluation', *BMJ*, 2001, vol. 322, pp. 1516–20

Buchbinder R, Jolley D, Wyatt M, '2001 Volvo Award Winner in Clinical Studies: Effects of a media campaign on back pain beliefs and its potential influence on management of low back pain in general practice', *Spine*, 2001, vol. 26, no. 23, pp. 2535–42

Buchbinder R, Staples M, Jolley D, 'Doctors with a special interest in back pain have poorer knowledge about how to treat back pain', *Spine*, 2009, vol. 34, no. 11, pp. 1218–26

Turner DJ, Xie W, Naylor JM, Harris IA, 'Strong versus weak opioids for post-discharge analgesia after surgery, a randomised trial', manuscript under review

Welch HG, Skinner JS, Schroeck FR, Zhou W, Black WC, 'Regional variation of computed tomographic imaging in the United States and the risk of nephrectomy', *JAMA Internal Medicine*, 2018, vol. 178, no. 2, pp. 221–27

Davenport R, 'Headache', *Practical Neurology*, 2008, vol. 8, pp. 335–43

Fisayo A, Bruce B, Newman NJ, Biousse V, 'Overdiagnosis of idiopathic intracranial hypertension', *Neurology*, 2016, vol. 86, pp. 341–50

Stunkel L, Kung NH, Wilson B, McClelland CM, Van Stavern GP, 'Incidence and causes of overdiagnosis of optic neuritis', *JAMA Ophthalmology*, 2018, vol. 136, no. 1, pp. 76–81

Pu Y, Mahankali S, J Hou J et al., 'High prevalence of pineal cysts in healthy adults demonstrated by high-resolution, noncontrast brain MR imaging', *American Journal of Neuroradiology*, 2007, vol. 28, no. 9, pp. 1706–709

'Pineal gland cysts: an evidence synthesis', Health Technology Assessment Unit, University of Calgary, 5 April 2016

6 Birth and death

Johansen R, Newburn M, MacFarlane A, 'Has the medicalisation of childbirth gone too far?', *BMJ*, 2002, vol. 324, pp. 892–95

Alfirevic Z, Devane D, Gyte GML, Cuthbert A, 'Continuous cardiotocography (CTG) as a form of electronic fetal monitoring (EFM) for fetal assessment during labour', *Cochrane Database of Systematic Reviews*, 2017, issue 2, article no. CD006066

Tan A, Schulze AA, O'Donnell CPF, Davis PG, 'Air versus oxygen for resuscitation of infants at birth', *Cochrane Database of Systematic Reviews*, 2005, issue 2, article no. CD002273

Jiang H, Qian X, Carroli G, Garner P, 'Selective versus routine use of episiotomy for vaginal birth', *Cochrane Database of Systematic Reviews*, 2017, issue 2, article no. CD000081

Viswanathan M, Hartmann K, Palmieri R et al., 'The use of episiotomy in obstetrical care: a systematic review: summary', 2005, *AHRQ Evidence Report Summaries*, Agency for Healthcare Research and Quality, Rockville, MD, 1998–2005

Boatin AA, Schlotheuber A, Betran AP et al., 'Within country inequalities in caesarean section rates: observational study of 72 low and middle income countries', *BMJ*, 2018, vol. 360, article no. k55

Human Reproduction Program, *WHO Statement on Caesarean Section Rates*, Department of Reproductive Health and Research, WHO, Geneva, 2015

World Health Organization, *WHO Recommendations: Intrapartum Care for a Positive Childbirth Experience*, WHO, Geneva, 2018

Einion AB, 'Women need more freedom during labour, not a medicalised birth script to follow', *The Conversation*, 8 March 2018, <https://theconversation.com/women-need-more-freedom-during-labour-not-a-medicalised-birth-script-to-follow-92079>

'National Core Maternity Indicators', Australian Institute for Health and Welfare, last updated 20 October 2020, <www.aihw.gov.au/reports/per/095/ncmi-data-visualisations/contents/labour-birth/b5>

Australian Institute of Health and Welfare, Peripartum hysterectomy in Australia: a working paper using the National Hospital Morbidity Database 2003–04 to 2013–14. Cat. no. PER 85, AIHW, Canberra, 2016

Frigerio M, Mastrolia SA, Spelzini F et al., 'Long-term effects of episiotomy on urinary incontinence and pelvic organ prolapse: a systematic review', *Archives of Gynecology and Obstetrics*, 2019, vol. 299, pp. 317–25

Begum T, Saif-Ur-Rahman KM, Yaqoot F et al., 'Global incidence of caesarean deliveries on maternal request: a systematic review and meta-regression', *BJOG*, 2021, vol. 128, pp. 798–806

Borges NC, de Deus JM, Guimarães RA et al., 'The incidence of chronic pain following Cesarean section and associated risk factors: a cohort of women followed up for three months', *PLOS ONE*, 2020, vol. 15, no. 9, article no. e0238634

Clark D, 'Between hope and acceptance: the medicalisation of dying', *BMJ*, 2002, vol. 324, no. 7342, pp. 905–907

QuickStats: Percentage distribution of deaths, by place of death – United States, 2000–2014. *MMWR Morbidity and Mortality Weekly Reports*, 2016, vol. 65, p. 357, <http://dx.doi.org/10.15585/mmwr.6513a6>

Doyle K, 'Out-of-hospital births on the rise in U.S.', *Scientific American*, 28 March 2016, <www.scientificamerican.com/article/out-of-hospital-births-on-the-rise-in-u-s>

Moskowitz EH, Nelson JL, 'The best laid plans', *Hastings Centre Report*, 1995, vol. 25, no. 6, pp. S3–5

Zhang B, Wright AA, Huskamp HA et al., 'Health care costs in the last week of life: associations with end-of-life conversations', *Archives of Internal Medicine*, 2009, vol. 169, no. 5, pp. 480–88

Ubel PA, Angott AM, Zikmund-Fisher BJ, 'Physicians recommend different treatments for patients than they would choose for themselves', *Archives of Internal Medicine*, 2011, vol. 171, no. 7, pp. 630–34

Clark D, 'Between hope and acceptance: the medicalisation of dying', *BMJ*, 2002, vol. 324, pp. 905–907

Kavalieratos D, Corbelli J, Zhang D et al., 'Association between palliative care and patient and caregiver outcomes', *JAMA*, 2016, vol. 316, no. 20, pp. 2104–14

Morris DB, *Illness and Culture in the Postmodern Age*, University of California Press, Berkley, 1998

Glazier RH, Dalby DM, Badley EM et al., 'Determinants of physician confidence in the management of musculoskeletal disorders', *Journal of Rheumatology*, 1996, vol. 23, pp. 351–56

Glazier RH, Dalby DM, Badley EM et al., 'Management of common musculoskeletal problems: a survey of Ontario primary care physicians', *Canadian Medical Association Journal*, 1998, vol. 158, pp. 1037–40

Cancer Australia, *Report on the Lung Cancer Screening Enquiry*, Cancer Australia, Sydney, 2020

7 Treating the problem

Aberegg SK, O'Brien JM Jr, 'The normalization heuristic: an untested hypothesis that may misguide medical decisions', *Medical Hypotheses*, 2009, vol. 72, no. 6, pp. 745–48

The NICE_SUGAR Study Investigators, 'Intensive versus conventional glucose control in critically ill patients', *New England Journal of Medicine*, 2009, vol. 360, pp. 1283–97

Kemp R, Prasad V, 'Surrogate endpoints in oncology: when are they acceptable for regulatory and clinical decisions, and are they currently overused?', *BMC Medicine*, 2017, vol. 15, article no. 134

Palmer SC, Saglimbene V, Mavridis D et al., 'Erythropoiesis-stimulating agents for anaemia in adults with chronic kidney disease: a network meta-analysis', *Cochrane Database of Systematic Reviews*, 2014, issue 12, article no. CD010590

References and further reading

Coyne DW, Goldsmith D, Macdougall IC, 'New options for the anemia of chronic kidney disease', *Kidney International Supplements*, 2017, vol. 7, no. 3, pp. 157–63

Little WC, Constantinescu M, Applegate RJ et al., 'Can coronary angiography predict the site of a subsequent myocardial infarction in patients with mild-to-moderate coronary artery disease?', *Circulation*, 1988, vol. 78, pp. 1157–66

Ambrose JA, Tannenbaum MA, Alexopoulos D et al., 'Angiographic progression of coronary artery disease and the development of myocardial infarction', *Journal of the American College of Cardiology*, 1988, vol. 12, no. 1, pp. 56–62

Al-Lamee R, Thompson D, Dehbi H-M et al., 'Percutaneous coronary intervention in stable angina (ORBITA): a double-blind, randomised controlled trial', *Lancet*, 2018, vol. 391, no. 10115, pp. 31–40

Boden WE, O'Rourke RA, Teo KK et al. for the COURAGE Trial Investigators, 'Optimal medical therapy with or without PCI for stable coronary disease', *New England Journal of Medicine*, 2007, vol. 356, pp. 1503–16

Sedlis SP, Hartigan PM, Teo KK et al. for the COURAGE Trial Investigators, 'Effect of PCI on long-term survival in patients with stable ischemic heart disease', *New England Journal of Medicine*, 2015, vol. 373, pp. 1937–46

Böhlke M, Barcellos FC, 'From the 1990s to CORAL (Cardiovascular Outcomes in Renal Atherosclerotic Lesions) Trial results and beyond: does stenting have a role in ischemic nephropathy?', *American Journal of Kidney Diseases*, 2015, vol. 65, pp. 611–22

Buchbinder R, Busija L, 'Why we should stop performing vertebroplasties', *Internal Medicine Journal*, 2019, vol. 49, pp. 1367–71

Ilic D, Neuberger MM, Djulbegovic M, Dahm P, 'Screening for prostate cancer', *Cochrane Database of Systematic Reviews*, 2013, issue 1, article no. CD004720

US Preventive Services Task Force, 'Screening for prostate cancer: US Preventive Services Task Force Recommendation Statement', *JAMA*, 2018, vol. 319, no. 18, pp. 1901–13

Pinsky PF, Prorok PC, Kramer BS, 'Prostate cancer screening – a perspective on the current state of the evidence', *New England Journal of Medicine*, 2017, vol. 376, pp. 1285–89

Echt DS, Liebson PR, Mitchell LB et al., 'Mortality and morbidity in patients receiving encainide, flecainide, or placebo – the Cardiac Arrhythmia Suppression Trial', *New England Journal of Medicine*, 1991, vol. 324, pp. 781–88

Poise Study Group, 'Effects of extended-release metoprolol succinate in patients undergoing non-cardiac surgery (POISE trial): a randomised controlled trial', *Lancet*, 2008, vol. 371, no. 9627, pp. 1839–47

Wiysonge CS, Bradley HA, Volmink J et al., 'Beta-blockers for hypertension', *Cochrane Database of Systematic Reviews*, 2017, issue 1, article no. CD002003

Aberegg SK, O'Brien JM, 'The normalization heuristic: an untested hypothesis that may misguide medical decisions', *Medical Hypotheses*, 2009, vol. 72, no. 6, pp. 745–48

The EC/IC Bypass Study Group, 'Failure of extracranial–intracranial arterial bypass to reduce the risk of ischemic stroke – results of an international randomized trial', *New England Journal of Medicine*, 1985, vol. 313, pp. 1191–1200

Goetzsche P, *Deadly Medicines and Organised Crime: How Big Pharma Has Corrupted Healthcare*, CRC Press, London, 2013

Prasad VK, Cifu AS, *Ending Medical Reversal: Improving Outcomes, Saving Lives*, Johns Hopkins University Press, Baltimore, 2015

Fleming TR, 'Surrogate endpoints and FDA's accelerated approval process', *Health Affairs*, 2005, vol. 24, no. 1, pp. 67–78

Kunnumakkara AB, Bordoloi D, Sailo BL, et al., 'Cancer drug development: the missing links', Exp Biol Med, 2019, vol.244, no. 8, pp. 663–689

Kim C, Prasad V, 'Strength of validation of surrogate endpoints used in the US Food and Drug Administration's approval of oncology drugs', Mayo Clin Proc 2016, vol. 91, pp. 713–25

Viswanathan M, Reddy S, Berkman N et al., 'Screening to prevent osteoporotic fractures: updated evidence report and systematic review for the US Preventive Services Task Force', *JAMA*, 2018, vol. 319, no. 24, pp. 2532–51

Morrisroe K, Nakayama A, Soon J et al., 'EVOLVE: the Australian Rheumatology Association's "top five" list of investigations and interventions doctors and patients should question', *Internal Medicine Journal*, 2018, vol. 48, pp. 135–43

George JN, Vesely SK, Woolf SH, 'Conflicts of interest and clinical recommendations: comparison of two concurrent clinical practice guidelines for primary immune thrombocytopenia developed by different methods', *American Journal of Medical Quality*, 2013, vol. 29, pp. 53–60

Buhagiar MA, Naylor JM, Harris IA et al., 'Effect of inpatient rehabilitation vs a monitored home-based program on mobility in patients with total knee arthroplasty: the HIHO randomized clinical trial', *JAMA*, 2017, vol. 317, no. 10, pp. 1037–46

Australian Private Hospitals Association, 'Knee surgery rehabilitation: new research not the whole story', media release, 15 March 2017, <phnews.org.au/knee-surgery-rehabilitation-new-research-not-the-full-story>

Levin D, Rao VM, 'Turf wars in radiology: updated evidence on the relationship between self-referral and the overutilization of imaging', *Journal of the American College of Radiology*, 2008, vol. 5, no. 7, pp. 806–10

Gazelle GS, Halpern EF, Ryan HS, Tramontano AC, 'Utilization of diagnostic medical imaging: comparison of radiologist referral versus same-specialty referral', *Radiology*, 2007, vol. 245, no. 2, pp. 517–22

Lungren MP, Amrhein TJ, Paxton BE et al., 'Physician self-referral: frequency of negative findings at MR imaging of the knee as a marker of appropriate utilization', *Radiology*, 2013, vol. 269, no. 3, pp. 810–15

Ma X, Wang H, Yang L, Shi L, Liu X, 'Realigning the incentive system for China's primary healthcare providers', *BMJ*, 2019, vol. 365, article no. l2406

Blumenthal D, Hsiao W, 'Lessons from the East – China's rapidly evolving health care system', *New England Journal of Medicine*, 2015, vol. 372, no. 14, pp. 1281–85

8 Prevention

Enright P, 'A homeopathic remedy for early COPD', *Respiratory Medicine*, 2011, vol. 105, pp. 1573–75

'Pharma watch: raising awareness or drumming up sales?', *Scientific American*, <www.scientificamerican.com/article/pharma-watch-raising-awareness-or-drumming-up-sales>

Lindsay GB, Merrill RM, Hedin RJ, 'The contribution of public health and improved social conditions to increased life expectancy: an analysis of public awareness', *Journal of Community Medicine and Health Education*, 2014, vol. 4, article no. 311

Centers for Disease Control and Prevention (CDC), 'Ten great public health achievements – United States, 1900–1999', *MMWR Morbidity and Mortality Weekly Report*, 1999, vol. 48, no. 12, pp. 241–43

Hunink MG, Goldman L, Tosteson AN et al., 'The recent decline in mortality from coronary heart disease, 1980–1990: the effect of secular trends in risk factors and treatment', *JAMA*, 1997, vol. 277, pp. 535–42

Goldman L, Cook EF, 'The decline in ischemic heart disease mortality rates: an analysis of the comparative effects of medical interventions and changes in lifestyle', *Annals of Internal Medicine*, 1984, vol. 101, pp. 825–36

GBD 2015 DALYs and HALE Collaborators, 'Global, regional, and national disability-adjusted life-years (DALYs) for 315 diseases and injuries and healthy life expectancy (HALE), 1990–2015: a systematic analysis for the Global Burden of Disease Study 2015', *Lancet*, 2016, vol. 388, no. 10053, pp. 1603–58

Helmuth L, 'Nine important things we've learned about the coronavirus pandemic so far', *Scientific American*, 5 September 2020, <www.scientificamerican.com/article/nine-important-things-weve-learned-about-the-coronavirus-pandemic-so-far>

Joyce M, 'Osteoporosis and vertebral compression fractures: advocacy groups and medical device maker spin misleading message', Healthnewsreview.org, 2 August 2018, <www.healthnewsreview.org/2018/10/osteoporosis-and-vertebral-compression-fractures-advocacy-groups-and-medical-device-maker-spin-misleading-message>

9 Medicalising normal

Tikkinen KAO, Leinonen JS, Guyatt GH et al., 'What is a disease? Perspectives of the public, health professionals and legislators', *BMJ Open*, 2012, vol. 2, article no. e001632

Erueti C, Glasziou P, Del Mar C, van Driel ML, 'Do you think it's a disease? A survey of medical students', *BMC Medical Education*, 2012, vol. 12, article no. 19

Epperson CN, Steiner M, Hartlage SA et al., 'Premenstrual dysphoric disorder: evidence for a new category for *DSM-5*', *American Journal of Psychiatry*, 2012, vol. 169, no. 5, pp. 465–75

Hantsoo L, Epperson CN, 'Premenstrual dysphoric disorder: epidemiology and treatment', *Current Psychiatry Reports*, 2015, vol. 17, no. 11, article no. 87

Ro C, 'The overlooked condition that can trigger extreme behaviour', BBC *Future*, 16 December 2019, <www.bbc.com/future/article/20191213-pmdd-a-little-understood-and-often-misdiagnosed-condition>

Khera R, Yuan L, Jiapeng L et al., 'Impact of 2017 ACC/AHA guidelines on prevalence of hypertension and eligibility for antihypertensive treatment in United States and China: nationally representative cross sectional study', *BMJ*, 2018, vol. 362, article no. k2357

Bell KJL, Doust J, Glasziou P, 'Incremental benefits and harms of the 2017 American College of Cardiology/American Heart Association high blood pressure guideline', *JAMA Internal Medicine*, 2018, vol. 178, no. 6, pp. 755–57

Xu Y, Wang L, He J et al., 'Prevalence and control of diabetes in Chinese adults', *JAMA*, 2013, vol. 310, no. 9, pp. 948–59

Cundy T, Ackermann E, Ryan EA, 'Gestational diabetes: new criteria may triple the prevalence but effect on outcomes is unclear', *BMJ*, 2014, vol. 348, article no. g1567

Vandorsten JP, Dodson WC, Espeland MA et al., 'NIH consensus development conference: diagnosing gestational diabetes mellitus', *NIH Consensus and State -of-the-Science Statements*, 2013, vol. 29, no. 1, pp. 1–31

Järvinen TLN, Michaëlsson K, Jokihaara J et al, 'Overdiagnosis of bone fragility in the quest to prevent hip fracture', *BMJ*, 2015, vol. 350, article no. h2088

Viswanathan M, Reddy S, Berkman N et al., 'Screening to prevent osteoporotic fractures: updated evidence report and systematic review for the US Preventive Services Task Force', *JAMA*, 2018, vol. 319, no. 24, pp. 2532–51

Kolata G, 'Bone diagnosis gives new data but no answers', *New York Times*, 28 September 2003, <www.nytimes.com/2003/09/28/us/bone-diagnosis-gives-new-data-but-no-answers.html>

Zhao J, Zeng X, Wang J, Liu L, 'Association between calcium or vitamin D supplementation and fracture incidence in community-dwelling older adults: a systematic review and meta-analysis', *JAMA*, 2017, vol. 318, no. 24, pp. 2466–82

Avenell A, Mak JCS, O'Connell D, 'Vitamin D and vitamin D analogues for preventing fractures in post-menopausal women and older men', *Cochrane Database of Systematic Reviews*, 2014, issue 4, article no. CD000227

Moynihan R, 'Caution! Diagnosis creep', *Australian Prescriber*, 2016, vol. 39, no. 2, pp. 30–31

Bi S, Klusty T, 'Forced sterilizations of HIV-positive women: a global ethics and policy failure', *AMA Journal of Ethics*, 2015, vol. 17, no. 10, pp. 952–57

Patel P, 'Forced sterilization of women as discrimination', *Public Health Reviews*, 2017, vol. 38, article no. 15

Gordon P, 'Is depression overdiagnosed? Yes', *BMJ*, 2007, vol. 335, p. 328

Whitely M, Raven M, '1 in 8 (over 3 million) Australians are on antidepressants – Why is the Lucky Country so miserable?', PsychWatch Australia, accessed 2 April 2021, <www.psychwatchaustralia.com/post/1-in-8-over-3-million-australians-are-on-antidepressants-why-is-the-lucky-country-so-miserable>

Healy D, *Let Them Eat Prozac*, New York University Press, New York, 2004

Goetzsche P, *Deadly Medicines and Organised Crime: How Big Pharma Has Corrupted Healthcare*, CRC Press, London, 2013

Cipriani A, Zhou X, Del Giovane C et al., 'Comparative efficacy and tolerability of antidepressants for major depressive disorder in children and adolescents: a network meta-analysis', *Lancet*, 2016, vol. 388, no. 10047, pp. 881–90

Sharma T, Guski LS, Freund N, Gøtzsche PC, 'Suicidality and aggression during antidepressant treatment: systematic review and meta-analyses based on clinical study reports', *BMJ*, 2016, vol. 352, article no. i65

Stevenson N, 'Autism doesn't have to be viewed as a disability or disorder', *The Guardian*, 16 July 2015, <www.theguardian.com/science/blog/2015/jul/16/autism-doesnt-have-to-be-viewed-as-a-disability-or-disorder>

Buchbinder R et al., Low Back Pain Series, *Lancet*, 2018, <www.thelancet.com/series/low-back-pain>

Bernstein DN, Brodell D, Li Y et al., 'Impact of the economic downturn on elective lumbar spine surgery in the United States: a national trend analysis, 2003 to 2013', *Global Spine Journal*, 2017, vol. 7, no. 3, pp. 213–19

Harris IA, Traeger A, Stanford R, Maher CG, Buchbinder R, 'Lumbar spine fusion: what's the evidence?', *Internal Medicine Journal*, 2018, vol. 48, no. 12, pp. 1430–34

Machado G, Lin C, Harris I, 'Spinal fusion surgery for lower back pain: it's costly and there's little evidence it'll work', *The Conversation*, 19 February 2018, <https://theconversation.com/spinal-fusion-surgery-for-lower-back-pain-its-costly-and-theres-little-evidence-itll-work-91829>

Harris IA, Dantanarayana N, Naylor JM, 'Spine surgery outcomes', *Australian and New Zealand Journal of Surgery*, 2012, vol. 82, pp. 625–29

Di Donato MF, Xia T, Iles R, Buchbinder R, Collie A, 'Patterns of opioid prescription and associated wage replacement duration in workers with accepted compensation claims for low back pain: a retrospective cohort study', *Pain*, 2021, manuscript under review

Blanchette MA, Rivard M, Dionne CE, Hogg-Johnson S, Steenstra I, 'Association between the type of first healthcare provider and the duration of financial compensation for occupational back pain', *Journal of Occupational Rehabilitation*, 2017, vol. 27, pp. 382–92

Webster BS, Bauer AZ, Choi YS et al., 'Iatrogenic consequences of early magnetic resonance imaging in acute, work-related, disabling low back pain', *Spine*, 2013, vol. 38, no. 22, pp. 1939–46

Emery DJ, Shojania KG, Forster AJ et al., 'Overuse of magnetic resonance imaging', *JAMA Internal Medicine*, 2013, vol. 173, no. 9, pp. 823–25

Foster NE, Koes B, Chou R et al., 'Prevention and treatment of low back pain: evidence, challenges, and promising directions', *Lancet*, 2018, vol. 391, no. 10137, pp. 2368–83

Rae T, Mitchell GK, Batstra L, 'Attention-deficit/hyperactivity disorder: are we helping or harming?', *BMJ*, 2013, vol. 347, article no. f6172

Paris J, Bhat V, Thombs B, 'Is adult attention-deficit hyperactivity disorder being overdiagnosed?', *Canadian Journal of Psychiatry*, 2015, vol. 60, no. 7, pp. 324–28

Waller A, Turon H, Mansfield E et al., 'Assisting the bereaved: a systematic review of the evidence for grief counselling', *Palliative Medicine*, 2015, vol. 30, no. 2, pp. 132–48

Frances A, 'Keith Connors, father of ADHD, regrets its current misuse: setting things straight on the ADHD diagnosis', *Psychology Today*, 28 March 2016, <www.psychologytoday.com/intl/blog/saving-normal/201603/keith-connors-father-adhd-regrets-its-current-misuse>

Schwartz A, *ADHD Nation: Children, Doctors, Big Pharma, and the Making of an American Epidemic*, Simon & Schuster, New York, 2016

Frances A, *Saving Normal: An Insider's Revolt Against Out-of-control Psychiatric Diagnosis, DSM-5, Big Pharma, and the Medicalization of Ordinary Life*, William Morrow & Co., New York, 2013

'Sarcopenia: new disease affects thousands', SBS News, 10 November 2016, <www.sbs.com.au/news/sarcopenia-new-disease-affects-thousands>

Joyner MJ, Paneth N, 'Promises, promises, and precision medicine', *Journal of Clinical Investigation*, 2019, vol. 129, no. 3., pp. 946–48

Gilbody S, Wilson P, Watt I, 'Benefits and harms of direct to consumer advertising: a systematic review', *BMJ Quality and Safety*, 2005, vol. 14, vol. 246–50

10 Healing

Choosing Wisely, '5 questions to ask your doctor or other health professional', <www.choosingwisely.org.au/resources/consumers/5-questions-to-ask-your-doctor>

Moynihan R, Sweet M, *Ten Questions You Must Ask Your Doctor: How to Make Better Decisions About Drugs, Tests and Treatments*, Allen & Unwin, Sydney, 2008

'Questions to ask your doctor', Healthdirect, <www.healthdirect.gov.au/questions-to-ask-your-doctor>

National Prescribing Service (NPS), 'Making wise choices about medicines', <www.nps.org.au/consumers/making-wise-choices-about-medicines>

Roozenbeek J, Schneider CR, Dryhurst S et al., 'Susceptibility to misinformation about COVID-19 around the world', *Royal Society Open Science*, 2020, vol. 7, article no. 201199

Institute of Medicine (US), *Roundtable on Value & Science-driven Health Care: Learning What Works: Infrastructure Required for Comparative Effectiveness Research: Workshop Summary*, National Academies Press, Washington, DC, 2011

Miller JD, 'Study affirms pharma's influence on physicians', *JNCI: Journal of the National Cancer Institute*, 2007, vol. 99, no. 15, pp. 1148–50

Engelberg, J, Parsons CA, Tefft J, 'Financial conflicts of interest in Medicine', SSRN, 2014, <https://ssrn.com/abstract=2297094>

Steinman MA, Shlipak MG, McPhee SJ, 'Of principles and pens: attitudes and practices of medicine housestaff toward pharmaceutical industry promotions', *American Journal of Medicine*, 2001, vol. 110, pp. 551–57

Doust J, Vandvik PO, Qaseem A et al., 'Guidance for modifying the definition of diseases. a checklist', *JAMA Internal Medicine*, 2017, vol. 177, no. 7, pp. 1020–25

Moynihan RN, Cooke GPE, Doust JA et al., 'Expanding disease definitions in guidelines and expert panel ties to industry: a cross-sectional study of common conditions in the United States', *PLOS Medicine*, 2013, vol. 10, no. 8, article no. e1001500

Donaldson MG, Cawthon PM, Lui L-Y et al., 'Estimates of the proportion of older white women who would be recommended for pharmacologic treatment by the new U.S. National Osteoporosis Foundation Guidelines', *Journal of Bone and Mineral Research*, 2009, vol. 24, no. 4, pp. 675–80

Nelson F, 'What do we mean when we call something a disease?', Medical Republic, 20 July 2018, <http://medicalrepublic.com.au/mean-call-something-disease/15737>

Saiz LC, Gorricho J, Garjón J et al., 'Blood pressure targets for the treatment of people with hypertension and cardiovascular disease', *Cochrane Database of Systematic Reviews*, 2018, issue 7, article no. CD010315

Tikkinen KAO, Leinonen JS, Guyatt GH et al., 'What is a disease? Perspectives of the public, health professionals and legislators', *BMJ Open*, 2012, vol. 2, article no. e001632

Flegal KM, Kit BK, Orpana H, Graubard BI, 'Association of all-cause mortality with overweight and obesity using standard body mass index categories: a systematic review and meta-analysis', *JAMA*, 2013, vol. 309, no. 1, pp. 71–82

Heath I, *The Mystery of General Practice*, Nuffield Provincial Hospitals Trust, London, 1995

Harris IA, Dao AT, 'Trends of spinal fusion surgery in Australia: 1997 to 2006', *Australia and New Zealand Journal of Surgery*, 2009, vol. 79, pp. 783–88

Harris I, Mulford J, Solomon M et al., 'Association between compensation status and outcome after surgery: a meta-analysis', *JAMA*, 2005, vol. 293, no. 13, pp. 1644–52

References and further reading

Shepstone L, Lenaghan E, Cooper C et al., 'Screening in the community to reduce fractures in older women (SCOOP): a randomised controlled trial', *Lancet* 2018, vol. 391, no. 10122, pp. 741–47

Verbeek JH, Martimo KP, Karppinen J et al., 'Manual material handling advice and assistive devices for preventing and treating back pain in workers', *Cochrane Database of Systematic Reviews*, 2011, issue 6, article no. CD005958

Beauchamp A, Batterham RW, Dodson S et al., 'Systematic development and implementation of interventions to Optimise Health Literacy and Access (Ophelia)', *BMC Public Health*, 2017, vol. 17, article no. 230

Austvoll-Dahlgren A, Oxman AD, Chalmers I et al., 'Key concepts that people need to understand to assess claims about treatment effects', *Journal of Evidence-Based Medicine*, 201, vol. 8, pp. 112–25

Bourne AM, Peerbux S, Jessup R et al., 'Health literacy profile of recently hospitalised patients in the private hospital setting: a cross sectional study', *BMC Health Services Research*, 2018, vol. 18, no. 1, article no. 877

Jessup RL, Osborne RH, Beauchamp A et al., 'Health literacy of recently hospitalised patients: a cross-sectional survey using the Health Literacy Questionnaire (HLQ)', *BMC Health Services Research*, 2017, vol. 17 article no. 52

Kelly PA, Haidet P, 'Physician overestimation of patient literacy: a potential source of health care disparities', *Patient Education and Counseling*, 2007, vol. 66, pp. 119–22

Main CJ, Buchbinder R, Porcheret M, Foster N, 'Addressing patient beliefs and expectations in the consultation', *Best Practice & Research Clinical Rheumatology*, 2010, vol. 24, no. 2-2, pp. 219–25

Hersch J, Barrat A, Jansen J et al., 'Use of a decision aid including information on overdetection to support informed choice about breast cancer screening: a randomised controlled trial', *Lancet*, 2015, vol. 385, no. 9978, pp. 1642–52

Tooke J, *Aspiring to Excellence: Final Report of the Independent Inquiry into Modernising Medical Careers*, MMC Inquiry, London, 2008

Best D, Lopes J, Pugh C, 'Re: "It's the duty of every doctor to get involved with research"', *BMJ*, 2015, vol. 351, article no. h6329

Ozdemir BA, Karthikesalingam A, Sinha S et al., 'Research activity and the association with mortality', *PLOS ONE*, 2015, vol. 10, article no. e0118253

Casarett D, 'The science of choosing wisely – overcoming the therapeutic illusion', *New England Journal of Medicine*, 2016, vol. 374, pp. 1203–205

'Choosing Wisely: a special report on the first five years 2017', Choosing Wisely, <www.choosingwisely.org/wp-content/uploads/2017/10/Choosing-Wisely-at-Five.pdf>

Brody H, 'Medicine's ethical responsibility for health care reform – the Top Five List', *New England Journal of Medicine*, 2010, vol. 362, no. 4, pp. 283–85

The Good Stewardship Working Group, 'The "Top 5" lists in primary care', *Archives of Internal Medicine*, 2011, vol. 171, no. 15, pp. 1385–90

O'Donnell J, 'The Kaiser Way: lesson for U.S. health care?', *USA Today*, 13 August 2014, <https://eu.usatoday.com/story/news/nation/2014/08/06/kaiser-permanente-obamacare-accountable-care-organizations-hospitals/12763591>

Abelson R, 'The face of future health care', *New York Times*, 20 March 2013, <www.nytimes.com/2013/03/21/business/kaiser-permanente-is-seen-as-face- of-future-health-care.html>

Wulff KC, Miller FG, Pearson SD, 'Can coverage be rescinded when negative trial results threaten a popular procedure? The ongoing saga of vertebroplasty', *Health Affairs*, 2011, vol. 30, pp. 2269–76

'Items which should not routinely be prescribed in primary care: guidance for CCGs', NHS Clinical Commissioners, London, 2017

Juch JNS, Maas ET, Ostelo RWJG et al., 'Effect of radiofrequency denervation on pain intensity among patients with chronic low back pain: the MINT randomized clinical trials', *JAMA*, 2017, vol. 318, pp. 68–81

Ozdemir BA, Karthikesalingam A, Sinha S et al., 'Research activity and the association with mortality', *PLOS ONE*, 2015, vol. 10, no. 2, article no. e0118253

Laliberte L, Fennell ML, Papandonatos G, 'The relationship of membership in research networks to compliance with treatment guidelines for early-stage breast cancer', *Medical Care*, 2005, vol. 43, no. 5. pp. 471–79

Wolfe SM, 'Does $760m a year of industry funding affect the FDA's drug approval process?', *BMJ*, 2014, vol./ 349, article no. g5012

Pham-Kanter G, 'Revisiting financial conflicts of interest in FDA advisory committees', *Milbank Quarterly*, 2014, vol. 92, no. 3, pp. 446–70

Pathirana T, Clark J, Moynihan R, 'Mapping the drivers of overdiagnosis to potential solutions', *BMJ*, 2017, vol. 358, article no. j3879

Nutbeam D, 'Health literacy as a public health goal: a challenge for contemporary health education and communication strategies into the 21st century', *Health Promotion International*, 2006, vol. 15, no. 3, pp. 259–67

Frakes MD, Gruber J, 'Defensive medicine: evidence from military immunity', NBER Working Paper No. 24846, National Bureau of Economic Research, Cambridge, MA, 2018

Bishop GF, Thomas RK, Wood JA, Gwon M, 'Americans' scientific knowledge and beliefs about human evolution in the year of Darwin', *National Center for Science Education*, 2010, vol. 30, no. 3, pp. 16–18, <https://ncse.com/library-resource/americans-scientific-knowledge-beliefs-human-evolution-year>

Gwon M, 'Measuring and understanding public opinion on human evolution', PhD thesis University of Cincinnati, 2012, <http://rave.ohiolink.edu/etdc/view?acc_num=ucin1353342586>

Kindig DA, Panzer AM, Nielsen-Bohlman L (eds), *Health Literacy: A Prescription to End Confusion*, National Academies Press, Washington, DC, 2004

Bauchner H, Fontanarosa PB, Thompson AE, 'Professionalism, governance, and self-regulation of medicine', *JAMA*, 2015, vol. 313, no. 18, pp. 1831–36

Stacey D, Légaré F, Lewis K et al., 'Decision aids for people facing health treatment or screening decisions', *Cochrane Database of Systematic Reviews*, 2017, issue 4, article no. CD001431

Colla CH, Kinsella EA, Morden NE et al., 'Physician perceptions of Choosing Wisely and drivers of overuse', *American Journal of Managed Care*, 2016. vol. 22, no. 5, pp. 337–43

Jones K, 'In whose interest? Relationships between health consumer groups and the pharmaceutical industry in the UK', *Sociology of Health & Illness*, 2008, vol. 30, pp. 929–43

Smith R, 'Medicine's need for philosophy', The BMJ Opinion (blog), 8 April 2016, <https://blogs.bmj.com/bmj/2016/04/08/richard-smith-medicines-need-for-philosophy>

Glasziou P, Sander S, Hoffmann T, 'Waste in COVID-19 research', *BMJ*, 2020, vol. 369, article no. m1847

References and further reading

Roozenbeek J, Schneider CR, Dryhurst S et al., 'Susceptibility to misinformation about COVID-19 around the world', *Royal Society Open Science*, 2020, vol. 7, article no. 201199

Madden DL, McLean M, Horton GL, 'Preparing medical graduates for the health effects of climate change: an Australasian collaboration', *Medical Journal of Australia*, 2018, vol. 208, pp. 291–92

Salas RN, Maibach E, Pencheon D et al., 'A pathway to net zero emissions for healthcare', *BMJ*, 2020, vol. 371, article no. m3785

Ivers N, Jamtvedt G, Flottorp S et al., 'Audit and feedback: effects on professional practice and healthcare outcomes', *Cochrane Database of Systematic Reviews*, 2012, issue 6, article no. CD000259

Badgery-Parker T, Pearson SA, Chalmers K et al., 'Low-value care in Australian public hospitals: prevalence and trends over time', *BMJ Quality and Safety*, 2019, vol. 28, pp. 205–14

Brehaut JC, Colquhoun HL, Eva KW et al., 'Practice feedback interventions: 15 suggestions for optimising effectiveness', *Annals of Internal Medicine*, 2016, vol. 164, pp. 435–41

Chalmers K, Badgery-Parker T, Pearson SA et al., 'Developing indicators for measuring low-value care: mapping Choosing Wisely recommendations to hospital data', *BMC Research Notes*, 2018, vol. 11, article no. 163

Chivian E, 'Why doctors and their organisations must help tackle climate change: an essay by Eric Chivian', *BMJ*, 2014, vol. 348, article no. g2407

Sainsbury P, Charlesworth K, Madden D et al., 'Climate change is a health issue: what can doctors do?', *Internal Medicine Journal*, 2019, vol. 49, pp. 1044–48

Talley NJ, 'A sustainable future in health: ensuring as health professionals our own house is in order and leading by example', *Medical Journal of Australia*, 2020, vol. 212, p. 344

Madden DL, Capon A, Truskett PG, 'Environmentally sustainable health care: now is the time for action', *Medical Journal of Australia*, 2020, vol. 212, pp. 361–62

Australian Medical Association, 'Environmental sustainability in health care – 2019', AMA, 20 March 2019, <https://ama.com.au/position-statement/environmental-sustainability-health-care-2019>

Doctors for the Environment Australia, 'An Australian Healthcare Sustainability Unit (HSU) – DEA proposal', <www.dea.org.au/wp-content/uploads/2021/01/DEA-HSU-Proposal-Final-.pdf>

Pencheon D, 'Developing a sustainable health care system: the United Kingdom experience', *Medical Journal of Australia*, 2018, vol. 208, pp. 284–85

Behavioural Economics Team of the Australian Government, 'Nudge vs superbugs: using behavioural economics to reduce the overprescribing of antibiotics', Department of the Prime Minister and Cabinet, 21 June 2018, <https://behaviouraleconomics.pmc.gov.au/projects/nudge-vs-superbugs-behavioural-economics-trial-reduce-overprescribing-antibiotics>

'Reducing musculoskeletal diagnostic imaging requests in general practice', Trial Review, Australian New Zealand Clinical Trial Registry, ACTRN 12619001503112, registered 31 October 2019, <www.anzctr.org.au/Trial/Registration/TrialReview.aspx?id=378625&isReview=true>

Acknowledgments

The book was written with the support of a Rockefeller Foundation Academic Writing Residency at the Bellagio Center in Italy. Our time spent at the center, and our interaction with the other residents, made the book a reality and enriched its content.

We would like to thank our co-workers and colleagues who have supported and encouraged our work. Thank you to our friends and colleagues Sherine Gabriel, Alexandra Barratt and Minna Johansson for allowing us to tell their stories. We would also like to acknowledge the excellent and professional support provided by our publisher with their editorial and general advice. We acknowledge, too, the support of our families and, specifically, the input from our partners (fellow doctors), who contributed to the initial discussions and editing (and provided the book title). They also allowed us the time we needed to write the book and indulged our need to endlessly discuss the book while on shared vacations. Thanks also to our extended families and friends, who gave us valuable feedback and advice during this journey.

Cartoon credits

Page 15 'First do no harm ...' by Benjamin Schwartz, published in *New Yorker*, 24 July 2017. *Cartoonstock*

Page 68 'One of us is a placebo ...' by David Banks. *Cartoonstock*

Page 96 'I can cure your back problem ...' by David Sipress, published in *New Yorker*, 2 June 2008. *Cartoonstock*

Page 118 'There's no easy way ...' by P.C. Vey, published in *New Yorker*, 30 June 2003. *Cartoonstock*

Page 162 'Nobody wants to hear ...' by Todd Condron. *Cartoonstock*

Page 203 'Oh darling ... what a pity ...' by Michael Leunig, courtesy of Michael Leunig.

Index

CPSIA information can be obtained
at www.ICGtesting.com
Printed in the USA
BVHW030247260322
632143BV00005B/19